PSYCHOSOMATIC
MEDICINE
A Practical Guide

Second Edition

PSYCHOSOMATIC MEDICINE
A Practical Guide

Second Edition

Michael Blumenfield, MD

*The Sidney E. Frank Professor Emeritus of Psychiatry
and Behavioral Sciences
New York Medical College
Valhalla, New York*

Maria Tiamson-Kassab, MD

*Assistant Clinical Professor of Psychiatry
New York Medical College
Consultation-Liaison Psychiatrist
VA Hudson Valley Health Care Systems
Castle Point, New York*

Wolters Kluwer | Lippincott Williams & Wilkins
Health
Philadelphia · Baltimore · New York · London
Buenos Aires · Hong Kong · Sydney · Tokyo

Acquisitions Editor: Charles W. Mitchell
Managing Editor: Sirkka E. Howes
Marketing Manager: Kimberly Schonberger
Manufacturing Manager: Ben Rivera
Project Manager: Nicole Walz
Design Coordinator: Doug Smock
Cover Designer: Andrew Gatto
Production Services: Laserwords Private Limited, Chennai, India

© 2009 by LIPPINCOTT WILLIAMS & WILKINS, a Wolters Kluwer business
530 Walnut Street
Philadelphia, PA 19106 USA
LWW.com

Library of Congress Cataloging-in-Publication Data
Blumenfield, Michael.
 Psychosomatic medicine : a practical guide / Michael Blumenfield, Maria Tiamson-Kassab.—2nd ed.
  p. ; cm.
 Rev. ed. of.: Consultation-Liaison Psychiatry: A Practical Guide/ [edited by] Michael Blumenfield, Maria L. A. Tiamson. c2003.
 Includes bibliographical references and index.
 ISBN-13: 978-0-7817-7242-6
 ISBN-10: 0-7817-7242-7
 1. Medicine, Psychosomatic. I. Tiamson-Kassab, Maria (Maria L. A.) II. Psychosomatic medicine. III. Title.
 [DNLM: 1. Psychosomatic Medicine—methods. 2. Psychophysiology. WM 90 B658p 2009]
 RC49.P822 2009
 616.08—dc22

                                                                    2008028640

Care has been taken to confirm the accuracy of the information presented and to describe generally accepted practices. However, the authors, editors, and publisher are not responsible for errors or omissions or for any consequences from application of the information in this book and make no warranty, expressed or implied, with respect to the currency, completeness, or accuracy of the contents of the publication. Application of the information in a particular situation remains the professional responsibility of the practitioner.

The authors, editors, and publisher have exerted every effort to ensure that drug selection and dosage set forth in this text are in accordance with current recommendations and practice at the time of publication. However, in view of ongoing research, changes in government regulations, and the constant flow of information relating to drug therapy and drug reactions, the reader is urged to check the package insert for each drug for any change in indications and dosage and for added warnings and precautions. This is particularly important when the recommended agent is a new or infrequently employed drug.

Some drugs and medical devices presented in the publication have Food and Drug Administration (FDA) clearance for limited use in restricted research settings. It is the responsibility of health care providers to ascertain the FDA status of each drug or device planned for use in their clinical practice.

To purchase additional copies of this book, call our customer service department at (800) 638-3030 or fax orders to (301) 223-2320. International customers should call (301) 223-2300.

Visit Lippincott Williams & Wilkins on the Internet: at WWW.LWW.com. Lippincott Williams & Wilkins customer service representatives are available from 8:30 AM to 6 PM, EST.

                                                      10 9 8 7 6 5 4 3 2 1

To our teachers, students, and patients who taught us all that we know.

With special thanks to Susan and Makhlouf for encouraging us to complete this project.

We would like to dedicate this second edition to all our colleagues who have brought the field of consultation-liaison psychiatry to subspecialty status and to the next generation of psychiatrists who will develop a new era in psychosomatic medicine.

Contents

Foreword

Consultation-Liaison Psychiatry: A Practical Guide comes at a crucial time in the history of both psychiatry and medicine. Modern medicine increasingly challenges the psychological equilibrium of patients. Both the sophisticated technology of the modern hospital and the multiple medicines and procedures that patients experience will foster both psychological and organic reactions that demand psychiatric assessment and treatment. Consultation-liaison psychiatry is the psychiatric subspecialty that links Psychiatry to the rest of Medicine. It is practiced both in hospital settings and outpatient arenas where the medically ill, or those who think they are medically ill, present to non-psychiatric physicians. This subspecialty has a unique body of knowledge. Its importance has been reified by the recent decision by the American Board of Psychiatry and Neurology to endorse Consultation-Liaison Psychiatry, to be labeled as Psychosomatic Medicine, for formal subspecialty status that will require both added fellowship training and a Board examination. There will never be enough formally trained consultation psychiatrists to meet the needs of patients or physicians who require such consultative services. Thus the general psychiatrist must possess a basic level of skills and knowledge to perform consultations and understand the stressors of specific diseases and treatments. They also need resources for this knowledge base. This volume clearly supplies such information.

Dr. Michael Blumenfield has been a leading consultation-liaison psychiatrist in practice, education and clinical research for over three decades. This book by him and his well respected co-author Dr. Maria Tiamson contains information that all psychiatrists will need on an ongoing basis, whatever their specialty may be. It offers a rapid introduction to the sophisticated advances in medicine that are increasingly seen in routine psychiatric practice. Special issues, such as transplant psychiatry, highly technical intensive care settings, and special problems with new drugs which foster organic reactions are discussed in a concise and clinically focused manner.

Each chapter outlines on the major clinical issues which the consulting psychiatrist will encounter. Much of the book is devoted to the psychiatric aspects of patients with neoplastic diseases, burn and traumatic injuries, cardiovascular states; chronic renal failure; and obstetrical problems. The significant incidence of psychiatric problems in these populations mandate collaborative care. Clinical pearls offer the reader advice on how to manage difficult comorbid clinical problems in each disease area. The patient vignettes in the chapters make them come alive. One of the most effective approaches to consultation psychiatry is to develop an ongoign relationship with a specific hospital unit or clinic. This has been termed "liaison" and allows an efficient manner to teach collegues about broad themes in managing psychiatric comorbidity as well as indirect supervision of problem cases. Drs. Blumenfield and Tiamson discuss the liaison potentials for working the interface of various specialized disease states. The strategy suggested for establishing such relationships will be useful to maximize the psychiatric interface with such settings.

Two chapters are of particular note. Dr. Michael Blumenfield is one of the leading experts on the psychological aspects of burn and trauma disorders. His prior book on the subject is well known to our field (1). Secondly, Dr. Tiamson has unique expertise on HIV/AIDS. This is an area where psychiatrists are increasingly called to manage both the demoralization often found in patients with such a disorder, as well as managing the psychological reactions to the medications and the disease, itself (2). As depression is increasingly recognized as a significant variable that predicts mortality both in myocardial infarction and cerebrovascular disease, the chapter on cardiology is essential for all psychiatrists. All psychiatrists must be familiar with the latest data in this area in order to better manage patients with cardiovascular disease. In addition to specific content areas, the initial chapter on performing the psychiatric consultation, as well as the concluding chapters on forensic aspects of consultation psychiatry and death and dying, are also important elements of consultation psychiatry but should be clearly within the skill set of general psychiatrists.

This volume provides a practical companion to psychiatrists entering the interface with medical and surgical conditions. It should be on the bookshelf of all psychiatrists since we are clearly physicians first and specialists second. The volume should also be part of the library of psychiatric nurses, social workers and psychologists who work in medical-surgical settings.

The experience of illness is one of life's great challenges. Psychiatrists can help individuals manage such events. This book will help in that task.

Thomas N. Wise, MD
Professor of Psychiatry & Behavioral Services
Johns Hopkins School of Medicine

REFERENCES

1. Blumenfield M and Schoeps M. *Psycholgoical Care of the Burn and Trauma Patient*. Baltimore: Williams & Wilkins, 1993.
2. Slavney PR. Diagnosing demoralization in consultation psychiatry. *Psychosomatics* 1999;40:325–329.

Preface

It has been 6 years since our first edition was published. We have been very gratified to see that students and housestaff as well as attendings, nurses and other mental health professionals working in the medical/surgical setting have found it useful to carry this book with them in their daily interactions with patients. In June 2003, Consultation/Liaison Psychiatry, now formally called *Psychosomatic Medicine*, was recognized as a subspecialty of Psychiatry with Board Certification by the American Board of Psychiatry and Neurology. This, of course, has heightened the interest in fellowships in this area after completion of psychiatry residencies. Not only does this bring more subspecialists into our field but also brings overall more interest in this area and greater expectations from our colleagues that these special topics will be addressed. There have been a few new large major textbooks in Psychosomatic Medicine, which includes the one edited by Blumenfield and Strain published by Lippincott with an accompanying DVD. The goal of this small textbook has been to be the first-line source of essential information as well as providing practical guidelines in the clinical approach to patients. Accessing the large major textbooks as well as up-to-date evidence-based research information obtained on the Internet should be the follow-up approach to clinical work.

For this edition we have reviewed each chapter and made additions or changes so that the topic is current and areas we had left out would be touched upon. Most of the practical guidelines are still quite applicable. We have added a separate chapter on Surgery and Transplant Psychiatry to consolidate the information on this topic. We have also created a special chapter on Women's Issues as well as one on Disaster Psychiatry. We tried to be consistent in this edition with regard to referring to consultation liaison psychiatry as C-L as compared to C/L viewing it as two components of the field rather than a dichotomy. In addition, we have revised some of the websites that are appropriate to each chapter. However, we recognize an Internet search, which can and should be conducted, will bring the most up-to-date information and can be specifically directed toward any pertinent questions.

We believe that in today's modern world it is incumbent on physicians to have access to the most up-to-date evidence-based research as well as a good working knowledge of the state of the art in approaching patients with a specific condition. In addition, the application of psychological insight and good clinical technique at the bedside is essential. We hope that this textbook will continue to be an important part of the mixture that clinicians will use along with the comprehensive textbooks and literature searches.

In addition, we want to remind you that direct communication and interaction with colleagues on the local level as well as at national meetings such as at the Academy of Psychosomatic Medicine and the American Psychiatric Association will round out the growth and continuous education that we all should pursue. As we move toward the second decade of this century, we will also have the opportunity to interact with bedside devices, which search the Internet and electronic records, with list serves between colleagues, with incorporation of video communication with colleagues and patients, and with many other new approaches that will be discussed in future renditions of this and other textbooks.

Michael Blumenfield, MD
Woodland Hills, California
Maria Tiamson-Kassab, MD
Castle Point, New York

Preface to the First Edition

As we survey the current Consultation-Liaison (C/L) Psychiatry scene, we have witnessed several major changes over the past two decades. At one time a large number of our patients were viewed as having very complex psychodynamic problems that interacted with their physical illness. Today, we more often see our patients as having problems that require delicate use of psychotropic medication along with skillful eclectic psychological support, including the newest behavioral-cognitive techniques.

In C/L training programs, it used to be common practice for trainees to engage in regular psychotherapy visits in the medical/surgical setting, which were supervised in leisurely teaching sessions. In many situations today, this has shifted to supervision on the fly, because attending physicians now carry busy clinical caseloads along with their supervisory responsibilities.

Previously, it had been more common for C/L psychiatrists, both trainees and attendings, to have regular liaison relationships with specific medical or surgical units where they would join work rounds a few times per week. Although such arrangements are not as widespread today, there are new opportunities for C/L psychiatrists to forge special relationships with newly developing specialty groups in areas such as AIDS, various transplant services, specialized oncology, trauma, fertility, high-risk obstetrics and others. At the end of each chapter of this book, we have made suggestions for potential areas of liaison activities. We believe that when it is possible to use this model, the most gratifying and effective work can be done.

We are ever impressed with the constant flow of new psychiatrists who are eager to step up to the plate and work at the interface between psychiatry and other specialties. As teachers in this field, it is always a privilege to work with our new colleagues at the bedside and see their empathy and sensitivity to patients. We welcome the opportunity to share their enthusiasm and pass on our experience in this work. There are certainly excellent textbooks in our specialty; we encourage our readers to build up a collection of them and to absorb their contents over time. It was not the purpose of this book to simply pull together the state of our knowledge in a comprehensive manner. Rather we hoped to provide an orientation to C/L psychiatry and to the major areas where it takes place. We drew upon our experience and our various lecture notes, which we have used over the past several years. We chose not to try to reference all this material since we knew we could not trace the sources of our own knowledge. We thank and appreciate our teachers and all the authors of textbooks and articles, which we have read and which continue to enrich our field.

We also appreciate that we are now working in an evidence-based medical environment. Modern psychiatrists must have the computer and the Internet as an extension of themselves. When we do our weekly sit-down chart rounds, we try to have someone checking the Internet as we review cases to keep us up to date on the latest literature. Ideally, appropriate print-outs should be incorporated into our consultation reports. Now with the development of wireless handheld devices, we expect that in a short time we shall be able to easily probe the literature as well as enter data and prepare our reports at the bedside.

We hope that this book not only will find its way into the pocket and be useful to both new and experienced C/L psychiatrists who take on the challenging and always inter-esting task of seeing patients at the medical/surgical interface, but also will be used by medical professionals in other spe-cialties. Many of our psychiatrist and psychologist colleagues who may work in our area or in another setting often have a profound interest and background in C/L psychiatry. We talk every day with nurses and social workers with whom we exchange insights about our mutual patients and who are quite tuned in to the concepts that we have discussed in this book. Whenever we encounter physical therapists, occupa-tional therapists, nutritionists, and other professionals who work with patients, there often is a curiosity mixed with an in-depth knowledge about these issues. Although we know that it is the rare non-psychiatric physician who will have the time to read our book, we do know that these pages are where they live. We also know that medical students who will go into every field of medicine have an enduring interest in what makes patients tick and especially how that interest relates to all aspects of medicine. So we hope this book will find its way into their curriculum and onto the desk and into the pockets of as many medical students as possible.

Michael Blumenfield, MD
Maria Tiamson, MD

Principles of
Consultation-Liaison
Psychiatry

Essential Concepts

- If possible, speak directly with medical staff and do a preliminary chart review before seeing the patient.
- Establish quick rapport with the patient by attending to physical comfort needs and by creating a private space within the hospital room.
- Assess carefully for potentially hidden suicidality, psychosis, and cognitive impairment.

Every 4 months, for many years, we have had the privilege of orienting a new group of psychiatry residents who are about to start their consultation-liaison (C-L) psychiatry or what is now known as *psychosomatic medicine rotation*. It will be their task to represent our service and hence our department to the rest of the medical center as they provide the initial response to requests for a psychiatric consultation. The residents have already had at least 2 years of psychiatric training and frequently it has been 3 years. They will have lots of backup and just about all of their cases will subsequently be seen face-to-face by an experienced supervisor with them at the bedside. They will also have an opportunity to discuss subsequent follow-up contact and any liaison work that may go on in the various medical/surgery services or that they may wish to develop during subsequent elective time with us.

This chapter and, in fact, the entire book consist of the specialized information and techniques that we try to provide for residents as they take on the task of being C-L psychiatrists or psychosomatic medicine specialists. We want them to be knowledgeable about psychosomatic medicine in each area in which they are called to consult. We hope this book will put us in the reader's pocket not so much as a detailed reference, but rather as preparation for the interesting and exciting world of psychosomatic medicine.

REQUEST FOR PSYCHIATRIC CONSULTATION

The initial request for a psychiatric consultation may come by phone to a secretary or by voice mail, fax, e-mail, page, or face-to-face personal contact. It is always preferable that the person requesting the consultation be the person who is clinically responsible for the care of the patient, usually the patient's physician. This is not always the case and, in some settings, a junior resident, medical student, nurse, social worker, administrator, or ward clerk may be designated to make contact with the psychiatrist or C-L service. There also should be a written indication in the chart that the responsible treating physician is aware of the consultation request and is in favor of it being carried out.

Usually the request for a consultation will include some indication of the urgency of the situation. In most acute care settings, a "stat" request means "as soon as possible," often within minutes or hours. Such urgent requests usually are best handled by a person-to-person contact. In acute hospital settings, most consultations are responded to within 24 hours. Depending on the situation, it may be perfectly acceptable to make initial contact with the patient within 48 to 72 hours, but we recommend checking in with the consultee, if the wait will be this long. Sometimes, we will make immediate contact with the patient to assess the urgency of the situation, provide a preliminary note in the chart, and indicate that we will be following up over the next few days.

BEFORE SEEING THE PATIENT

We recommend that you speak with the requesting physician before seeing the patient. Depending on the case, it may be appropriate to ask for the patient's prognosis, planned surgery, planned discharge, medications, indication of perceived danger, whether the patient knows you are coming, and you cannot go wrong with, "Is there anything else I should know?"

On arriving at the hospital unit, take advantage of the opportunity to speak with the nurse or social worker who is working with the patient. Although rules of confidentiality may prevent you from revealing everything you know about the patient to others, it is always fair game to listen to any information provided by others who know the patient. Do not forget to talk to any person who is assigned to be on "one-on-one" or "special" or "constant observation."

A family member will often be at the bedside when you arrive. Family often will be eager to speak with you, which is entirely appropriate. Although the patient may indicate that he or she would like family to be present during your interview, we recommend that you have at least some private time with your patient. This will allow sensitive or embarrassing issues to be more freely divulged. Therefore, when you arrive at the bedside to introduce yourself, it is usually best for you to politely indicate that you would like to speak with the patient privately and that this is your usual method of consultation. Most people will understand and accept it. After you have held a private interview, you can ask your patient's permission to speak with a family member and, depending on the circumstances, offer to keep the content of your interview confidential. You also should ask your patient's permission to contact an outside psychiatrist or other mental health professional that he or she has worked with. If the patient is too confused or psychotic to provide this permission, the medical urgency of the situation usually allows you to legally pursue such information anyway.

Problems that commonly lead to requests for psychiatric consultation in the medical/surgical setting are outlined in Table 1.1.

REVIEWING THE CHART

We recommend that you review the hospital chart before seeing the patient. This review may be more or less thorough or time-consuming, depending on the clinical question. There are two important facts of which you should be aware in regard to reviewing the chart. First, as a participant now in the care of the patient, you are responsible for the contents of the chart. Second, you will be lucky if you can decipher half of the handwritten notes!

The approach to the review of the chart is an art. Some people will start with the last progress notes, others will first look at the admitting notes, and still others will look initially at the most recent laboratory data or the nurse's notes. In reality, it is usually necessary to read all of the above-mentioned data, as a bare minimum in any chart review. In addition, glance at the medication list as well. Sometimes there will be an

TABLE 1.1. Problems that Commonly Lead to Requests for Psychiatric Consultation in the Medical/Surgical Setting

1. Acute stress reactions
2. Aggression or impulsivity
3. Agitation
4. Acquired immunodeficiency syndrome or humanimmuno-deficiency virus infection
5. Alcohol and drug abuse (including withdrawal states)
6. Anxiety or panic
7. Assessment of psychiatric history
8. Burn sequelae
9. Change of mental status
10. Child abuse
11. Coping with illness
12. Death, dying, and bereavement
13. Delirium
14. Dementia
15. Depression
16. Determination of capacity and other forensic issues
17. Eating disorders
18. Electroconvulsive therapy
19. Ethical issues
20. Factitious disorders
21. Family problems
22. Geriatric abuse
23. Hypnosis
24. Malingering
25. Pain
26. Pediatric psychiatric illness
27. Personality disorders
28. Posttraumatic stress disorder
29. Pregnancy-related care
30. Psychiatric care in the intensive care unit
31. Psychiatric manifestations of medical and neurological illness
32. Psychological factors affecting medical illness
33. Psychological and neuropsychological testing
34. Psycho-oncology
35. Psychopharmacology of the medically ill
36. Psychosis
37. Restraints

TABLE 1.1. *Continued*

---

38. Sexual abuse
39. Sleep disorders
40. Somatoform disorders
41. Suicide
42. Terminal illness
43. Transplantation issues

(From Bronheim HE, Fulop G, Kunkel EJ, et al. The Academy of Psychosomatic Medicine practice guidelines for psychiatric consultation in the general medical setting. *Psychosomatics* 1998;39(4):8–30, with permission.)

off-service note or even a complete summary by another consultant to bring you up to speed. After you interview the patient, you will have a much better idea of which information is most relevant.

APPROACH TO THE PATIENT

Psychiatrists frequently do not wear white coats when working in their offices. However, in the medical/surgical setting, we suggest that "when in Rome do as the Romans do." If the other physicians usually wear white coats, we think it is a good idea that the C-L consultant does likewise. This clearly identifies your medical background and, in most cases, contributes to making the patient more comfortable with your visit.

Although it seems quite basic, you should knock on the door and give the patient a chance to acknowledge that you are entering the room. If the patient is in the midst of a procedure or is in the bathroom or being bathed, it is only proper to announce that you regret the interruption and that you will be back. If the patient is on the telephone, eating, or having visitors, we suggest that you tactfully indicate who you are and that you would like to speak with him or her. Most patients will agree happily to interrupt their activity or visit to speak to you.

If the patient shares a room, you can ask the roommate to please step into a different part of the unit so that you can have a private interview. However, in most cases, this is not possible, and you will have to resort to techniques like drawing the curtains, speaking softly, and perhaps turning up or down the nearby radio or television to facilitate the interview and yet make it as private as possible.

In the ideal situation, the patient would have been briefed about your impending visit by the treating physician and therefore will not be surprised when you appear. Unfortunately, this is not always the case. When you enter, identify yourself by name and mention that you are a psychiatrist. Depending on the circumstances, you can and should add information that explains that you are part of the treatment team, that you see all or most of the patients in that particular unit (e.g., burn, transplant, or dialysis). It may be useful to mention that the patient's doctor has specifically asked you to see him or her. If you have reason to believe that the patient does not expect you and or may be resistant to your visit, it may be helpful to have one of the treating physicians or nurses actually introduce you to the patient.

If the patient says that he or she does not want to talk with you, you will need to assess the clinical situation to determine how important it is for you to gain your patient's cooperation. Simply repeating that the patient's doctor has asked you to speak with him or her and that he or she does not have to say anything that he or she does not want to share can sometimes overcome this resistance. If the psychiatric issue is not urgent (e.g., evaluation of a long-standing nonsuicidal depression), there is no need to persist. The patient may or may not be agreeable to your return at a later time. However, if the situation is an emergency (e.g., acute suicidality or a life-threatening alcohol withdrawal), you should insist upon seeing the patient. It is not unusual for the patient to be upset because he or she has to be evaluated by a psychiatrist (i.e., "I'm not crazy! Why should I see you?"). An approach would be as follows: "Mr. Smith, I don't just see mentally disturbed patients. Besides, no one has said that you are crazy. I deal with medically ill patients who do not necessarily have psychiatric history, but who have some issues dealing with their illness. I hope to be able to be of help to you." Sometimes you can use the patient's desire to leave the hospital as leverage: "Unfortunately, Mr. Smith, before you can leave the hospital I will have to do a psychiatric assessment to make sure you will be safe at home." In all cases where there is resistance to you seeing the patient or where you are limited in your ability to do a proper consultation, you should document this in the chart and notify the treating physician immediately.

When you cannot speak the patient's language, a competent translator is obviously required. Generally speaking, we recommend that the translator not be a close family member or friend because this may inhibit your patient from revealing important aspects of his or her history. Of course, in many situations, the family member will know all the details of the case and this will not be a problem. In working with translators, we usually ask that they translate exactly what we say and exactly what the patient answers, to minimize the addition of personal opinions or impressions into the translation. However, when there are cultural issues, which may be influencing the clinical picture, there is nothing wrong with asking the translator if you are missing any significant issues or if he or she has an opinion about what the patient is really trying to communicate.

THE SPANISH-SPEAKING AMPUTEE

A 24-year-old Spanish-speaking man was interviewed with a translator after surgery. He had an amputation of his right lower leg 6 months after a motor vehicle accident and several failed surgeries to save his leg. On the basis of the history and mental status, the impression of the consultant was that the patient had come to accept that he would be better off with a prosthesis. The patient appeared to be mildly depressed, denied any suicidal ideation, and had agreed to come for some outpatient follow-up. However, the translator seemed to be very concerned when he realized that the patient was going to be discharged to his home. The consultant noted that the translator appeared upset and when he asked him the reason, the translator explained that he was from the same country as the patient and knew the rural area where the patient was raised. He told the psychiatrist that he was almost sure that the patient would kill himself. He explained that, for this patient living without his leg meant he was no longer macho and that he could not picture himself ever being a functioning male again. A Spanish-speaking psychiatrist was located who confirmed that there were these deep-seated feelings, including suicidal intent. The patient was briefly hospitalized in a psychiatric unit. He was treated with short-term psychotherapy, which included educational material about prostheses and a visit by a Spanish-speaking patient who also had a prosthesis. The patient was subsequently discharged to outpatient care.

THE INTERVIEW

We are assuming that the reader of this book has had training and experience in both a medical interview of a physically ill or injured patient, as well as experience and expertise in doing a psychiatric interview that would include a mental status evaluation. The interview required in the C-L setting is a hybrid of both.

After a proper introduction and the establishment of as confidential a setting as possible, we often make an effort to attend to the patient's physical comfort. Although offering the patient a drink of water, adjusting the bed, or untangling IV lines may be symbolic in nature, these can go a long way toward demonstrating that you care about the patient. It is also important that you make yourself comfortable by finding a place to sit down, preferably in a chair rather than on the patient's bed.

Your opening statement will vary with the circumstances, but it will probably be some variation of, "Can you tell me what brought you to the hospital?" You may have preceded this with, "Your doctor has told me something about your situation, but I would like to hear about it from you." Some situations (e.g., when the patient is acting in an agitated or tearful manner or is perhaps wanting to sign out against medical advice from the hospital) call for a completely different approach. In such a case, it usually will be best to acknowledge that you understand that there is a problem and that you would like to hear about it from the patient.

When dealing with confused or overtly psychotic patients, the opening approach also will have to be adjusted. They may not grasp that you are a psychiatrist and that you are there to evaluate them. You will need to be brief and directive because their attention span may not allow for a complete interview and for the development of rapport between you and the patient. One other situation will dictate the nature of the interview from the very beginning and that is when the patient is in severe pain. Pain trumps all! This means that when the patient is obviously in significant pain, it is usually best that you turn your attention to the nature of the pain, location, duration, and intensity and try to understand what makes it better or worse. A major part of such a consultation is going to be to determine whether the patient is undermedicated for pain and you are losing no ground if you do that first. Your interest and concern in this area will allow you to proceed with other parts of the interview later.

After the opening question, you should try to move into the listening mode. Experienced interviewers know that some of the most valuable information is going to come in response to this initial question. In general, the approach of using open-ended questions first, followed up by more specific questions, will work well. Keep in mind that it will probably be useful for you to hear firsthand about the medical/surgical problem, but, in most cases, there is no need for you to meticulously develop each medical symptom, which has already been done. On the other hand, you do not want to go straight into a psychiatric interview, because the patient, in most cases, did not come to the hospital for this type of care and is likely preoccupied with the medical/surgical issues. You will need to learn to weave the medical and psychiatric interview together, ultimately in a seamless manner. Ideally, your bridges to psychological issues and mental status will be the patient's associations, which will allow you to cross over spontaneously at the time the patient brings them up or when you return to them at a later point. There is no one way to conduct an interview in the medical/surgical setting. In addition to an assessment of the consultation question that you have been asked and an understanding of the patient's main concern, there are four areas about which you should obtain basic information. These areas are as follows:

- Mood and affect
- Suicidality
- Psychosis
- Cognitive functioning

There also should be at least a brief assessment for a variety of psychiatric conditions, such as substance abuse, domestic violence, obsessive compulsive disorder (OCD), panic, or other anxiety disorders.

An initial consultation usually is done in the first visit, which means that you obtain the essential information to write your consultation report and recommendations. However, there are circumstances, particularly when the patient is very ill, not cooperative, or when the patient or the interviewer has to leave, in which a repeat meeting or meetings will be required before an adequate consultation report can be made. A note should be written in the chart at the time of any patient contact, even when the interview is truncated for some reason.

As mentioned earlier, it is not our purpose in this chapter to teach you how to do a proper interview, but we recommend that you read Dr. Daniel Carlat's *Practical Guide on the Psychiatric Interview* (Lippincott Williams & Wilkins, 2005) for this purpose. However, we do want to highlight some of the components of the interview (discussed in subsequent chapters) that often become a central focus of the C-L interview.

Mood and Affect

Evaluate both the patient's mood and affect (the outward expression of mood). Any loss of health or function usually is accompanied by depressive symptoms. Evaluation of the significance of these symptoms is complicated by the presence of physical illness, which frequently brings with it poor appetite, sleep difficulty, and sometimes apathy and withdrawal. Low self-esteem and self-worth are helpful clues for depression in the medically ill. Ask also about previous clinical depression and family history of affective disorders, both of which should alert you to the possibility of current depression. Pay careful attention to the time sequence of the depressive symptoms in relation to the onset of physical illness and the initiation of medications, because certain disease states and drugs can cause depression. Ask about any past episodes of mania that would suggest bipolar disorder. The experienced interviewer will know that such questions also should describe the behavior you are looking for, rather than only asking if the patient had a particular mood. These include asking about spending sprees, decreased need for sleep, promiscuity, and other manic-type behaviors.

Suicidality

Assessment of suicidality is an essential part of any interview. Do not neglect it in the medical setting because of a misguided concern that such questions will upset the patient. One good question that can lead gently into the topic of suicidality is, "Do you ever feel like giving up?" An affirmative answer should be followed up by asking what kind of thoughts go through the patient's mind and eventually asking if the patient has any thoughts about wanting to kill himself or herself. Even a negative response to the lead-in question ultimately should be followed up with a clear question as to whether the patient is having any suicidal ideas at present. Experienced interviewers will develop their own techniques for suicide assessment. It can be done in an empathic caring manner, which will usually be accepted by the patient. The results of this assessment will affect disposition and will, of course, determine if the patient may need to be transferred to a psychiatric facility.

Psychosis

Our medical/surgical colleagues may pick up the presence of psychosis, which they may recognize as such or as aberrant or unacceptable behavior that causes treatment noncompliance. In your assessment of psychosis, you will need to determine whether this is a symptom of recent onset or part of a preexisting psychiatric disorder, such as schizophrenia. You also will need to consider the possibility that the psychotic symptoms may in fact be related to a medical condition. Visual, olfactory, and tactile hallucinations, for example, often are caused by an organic or medical condition. There are also many medications and drug interactions, as well as substances of abuse, that can result in psychotic symptoms. The experienced C-L consultant eventually will become familiar with most of these interactions. It is important that even a basic interview screens for psychotic manifestation in some depth.

Cognition

The C-L consultant must search for the most subtle disturbance in cognition. While you obtain the history, listen carefully for evidence of difficulty in word finding, concentration, or disorientation. Although you can get a pretty good impression of cognition during the course of getting a history, it is usually a good idea to ask some formal questions to evaluate cognition. Ask the patient to subtract backward by sevens, starting with 100, or to do simple calculations, such as, "how many nickels in $1.10?" This is a good test of concentration. To test short-term memory, ask your patient to repeat three unrelated nouns, such as "blue, peanut butter, and elephant" and ask him or her to repeat the objects 5 minutes later. Asking the patient to spell a word, such as "world" or "horse," (forward and backward) is also a good quick test of concentration. All of these tasks are best considered screening tests, and poor performance may be a function of poor academic achievement or anxiety and should be followed up with further clinical evaluation.

We also recommend some easily administered paper and pencil tests, such as the draw-a-clock test. Give your patient a piece of paper and a pencil and ask him or her to draw the face of a clock, with numbers and hands in the position of 10 minutes after 8 o'clock. This will test memory and the ability to handle spatial relations. The most commonly used assessment instrument is the Mini Mental State Examination (MMSE), which allows the computation of a score from 0 to 30. This measure of cognitive functioning is repeated and followed over the course of the hospitalization. If there are cognitive deficits, you need to determine the underlying etiology. Chapter 10 provides a suggested approach to this workup.

In addition to the screening tools mentioned in the preceding text, there are some brief depression inventories [e.g., Hamilton Depression Rating Scale (Ham-D) or Zung Depression Scale], as well as two popular screening tools, CAGE and the Michigan Alcoholism Screening Test (MAST), which are used to assess alcoholism. These tools are used sometimes as part of the consultation.

You will usually rely on the physical examination of the treating physician to provide information on the physical state of the patient, along with laboratory and other tests. There may be times, however, when you will want to do a limited physical examination. This may include organ-specific evaluations for unexplained somatic complaints or check for medication side effects (i.e., cog wheeling), observable signs of self-injury, intravenous drug abuse, or the presence of frontal release signs, tremor, and parkinsonian symptoms.

There are many other things that need to be evaluated during the course of your interview with the patient, which will be discussed in later chapters. We mention three of them at this point because they so frequently have great significance and yet often are neglected until they rear their heads as major problems.

1. **Pain and pain management**. It is important to hear out the patient on how much pain he or she is having and whether the pain management appears to be adequate (Chapter 14).
2. **Thoughts about dying**. This is a sensitive topic for many people, but if asked in a matter-of-fact manner, patients may share fears, anxieties, and concerns and gain great comfort in doing so (Chapter 19).
3. **Fantasies about why and how the patient became sick or was injured**. Allowing your patients to share their thoughts and feelings about their illness will provide you with insight into their day-by-day struggles (Chapter 16).

THE CONSULTATION NOTE

Once you have reviewed the chart, obtained any necessary information from collateral sources, and interviewed the patient, you have to write a note in the chart. This is a very important note, which will be read by hospital personnel and can be reviewed by hospital review committees, as well as insurance and managed care companies. A court can subpoena it and medical records are legally available to patients. However, most important is the fact that the consultation note will be read and used by the treating physicians and nurses in the care of the patient.

SAMPLE CONSULTS

The following are sample consultations reconstructed from our files. There is no one style to which a note must conform. So much will depend on the particular circumstances of the case, as well as the usual practices of the doctor, service, and hospital. As you can see, these consultations are not all the same style and have been written by different people.

CASE 1

The patient is a 56-year-old woman with an 8-month history of ovarian cancer. She was treated by surgery and chemotherapy. She was hospitalized on (date) with plans to undergo a second round of chemotherapy. The routine medical workup was in progress when the patient abruptly told the nurse that she was going to leave the hospital and wanted her clothes. Review of the hospital chart revealed that the patient was currently on Prozac 20 mg, prescribed by her internist shortly after she was diagnosed with cancer. She has not seen a psychiatrist or other mental health professional.

The patient was initially reluctant to talk to a psychiatrist, but after a few minutes she was quite cooperative. She appeared anxious and acknowledged that she was fearful of dying in the hospital. She said that she had been told that she would only have to be in the hospital overnight and became upset when she found out that the doctors anticipated that the hospital stay would have to be several days longer. When she gets anxious, she describes episodes of palpitations and a "terrible feeling in the pit of my stomach." She has had similar feelings in the past (when her mother died) and more recently when she was told of the diagnosis of cancer. During the latter time, she had crying episodes with difficulty sleeping on and off for about 3 months. She believes that the Prozac was helpful for these symptoms, although her anxiety has continued. The patient also revealed that her mother died of lung cancer at the age of 57 years and the patient's fifty-seventh birthday is next week. The patient and her husband are both high school teachers. She has been married for 32 years and has two grown sons (ages 29 and 31 years) who are single, live out of the home, and are in the computer business. She describes her family as very close and supportive, but that she can't talk with them about her worries about her illness because they only insist that she is going to be fine.

Mental Status Exam: The patient related in a very intense manner. Her speech was relevant and coherent. Her mood was anxious and she would become tearful and depressed when talking about her mother. She showed a full range of affect, which was appropriate to content and situation. She said she slept poorly and needed sleeping pills (Ambien 5 mg) to fall asleep and sometimes would feel that she was up most of the night. Sometimes she had nightmares, but can't recall the content and isn't sure if they wake her up. She denied suicidal ideation and expressed fear that she was going to die when she turned 57 years old, the age that her mother died of lung cancer. There is no evidence of auditory or visual hallucinations, paranoid ideation, or overt psychosis. The patient was oriented in all three spheres and could spell the word "world" forward and backward. She performed serial sevens adequately and recalled three objects within 5 minutes. When it was suggested to her that her anxiety was intensifying because she was approaching her fifty-seventh birthday, which was the age that her mother died, she readily agreed, demonstrating some insight into her concerns. She accepted the idea that she should stay in the hospital for a few more days for her treatment. Overall her judgment seemed good.

Impression:

1. Adjustment reaction with anxiety and depression
2. Nemesis complex (patient expecting to die at age 57 years, as did her mother)

Recommendation:

1. Continue Prozac 20 mg per day
2. Add Klonopin 0.5 mg twice a day (b.i.d.) by mouth (po)

3. *I will follow her in regular psychotherapy visits during this hospitalization*
4. *Patient is receptive to outpatient referral for psychiatric follow-up*
5. *We have also set up at the patient's request for a joint meeting with the husband to explain the treatment plan (this will take place tomorrow)*
6. *I have discussed this consultation with Dr. X, the referring physician*

John Smith, MD
Beeper #1234
Tel #5678

CASE 2

The patient is a 35-year-old male who is HIV-positive. He was recently discharged after an anaphylactic reaction to antibiotics. The patient has been exhibiting acute mental status changes for the past few days. The patient has a history of depression and anxiety, as well as polysubstance dependence. His HIV is asymptomatic. He has an undetectable viral load and a CD4 count of 300. A week ago, the patient developed a high-grade fever and malaise. He was seen by his doctor and placed on antibiotics, after which he developed rashes all over his body. He was hospitalized briefly and discharged. Shortly after he came home, his wife states that he was acting strangely. He walked around the house with two different colored socks and wore his shorts inside out. His family initially thought that he was kidding around. He also started asking weird questions, which alarmed his wife and prompted her to take him to the emergency room (ER).

At the ER, the patient became combative and belligerent, refusing to cooperate with any of the doctors. He had to be restrained and a psychiatric consultation was requested. Labs could not be drawn.

When seen, the patient was very agitated, despite having received lorazepam (2 mg IM) and being placed in four-point restraints. He was oriented to his first name and not his last. He thought he was in his father's house. He was not oriented to day and date, but he knew the year. He was screaming at staff and demanding to get out of restraints. He was very distractible and unable to focus on the questions asked. A complete mental status exam was not possible, as the patient was severely agitated and uncooperative.

A review of his old record revealed that he is on methadone (80 mg per day), sertraline (100 mg per day), and clonazepam (2 mg per day). He is also on antiretroviral therapy, which included Zerit, Epivir, and Viracept.

Impression: Delirium, etiology to be determined [?encephalitis, ?meningitis, ?drug-induced, ?other central nervous system (CNS) pathology]

Recommendation:

1. *Complete blood count (CBC), blood chemistry panel, vitamin B-12, and folate*
2. *Toxicology screen*
3. *Computerized tomography (CT) of the head*
4. *Lumbar puncture (LP)*
5. *Neurology consult*
6. *Continue four-point restraints for safety of patient and others*
7. *Constant observation for self-destructive behavior*
8. *Haloperidol (2 mg every 4 hours) when necessary (PRN), with lorazepam (2 mg every 4 hours) when necessary for severe agitation*
9. *We will follow the patient closely with you. Thank you for the consult*

Mary Smith, MD
Beeper #1234
Tel #5678

Psychocardiology

Essential Concepts

- Patients having a first heart attack almost always deny that their symptoms are cardiac in origin.
- Depression and other acute emotional stress can precipitate acute cardiac symptoms and, in some cases, may be responsible for sudden death.
- Panic disorder is often misdiagnosed as cardiac disease, causing patients to get million-dollar workups before the true meaning is understood.
- Delirium is a very common psychiatric complication of coronary artery bypass graft (CABG) surgery.
- Psychotropic medications can cause cardiac side effects, but physicians should not be afraid to use them.

Heart disease is one of the best examples of the mind–body interaction. In every aspect of cardiovascular illness, it is relatively easy to discern the dynamic interplay that occurs between all the components of the biopsychosocial equation. Cardiologists and psychiatrists need to be aware that the onset, manifestation, and progress of cardiovascular conditions are influenced by underlying psychological issues. Conversely, a person's mental state is affected by the presence of cardiovascular disease and the treatment for it.

PSYCHOLOGICAL FACTORS AND THE HEART

Anxiety and the Heart

Every medical student knows that stress and anxiety cause a transient increase in heart rate and blood pressure. It is also established that atrial and even ventricular arrhythmias can occur during psychological stress in people who have underlying cardiac pathology. Stress induced by public speaking or mental arithmetic tasks has been shown to induce abnormal heart wall motion in susceptible people. There are two possible mechanisms for stress-induced cardiac arrhythmia: (1) vagal stimulation may directly cause heart rate variability and (2) autonomic arousal may cause increased catecholamines, which may act either directly on the myocardium or indirectly, by causing hypertension.

In addition to causing cardiac arrhythmias, anxiety also may play a role in coronary artery disease (CAD). Animal research has shown that increased sympathetic activity due to stress can promote atherogenesis. Norepinephrine and epinephrine effects on arterial tone can cause coronary spasms, as well as rupture of atherosclerotic plaques. Mental stress, especially anger, has been shown to decrease platelet stickiness and may even cause narrowing of the arteries.

A panic attack is a common psychiatric manifestation (Table 2.1). Patients having a panic attack frequently present with chest pain, shortness of breath, and other classically "cardiac" symptoms. Chest pain is a difficult symptom to interpret because it can signal true cardiac disease, a panic attack, or both. Psychiatrists tend to get involved in two different scenarios: (1) true cardiac disease with denial and (2) panic attack that masks as cardiac disease.

Typically, a patient experiencing a first episode of true cardiac chest pain will use the defense mechanism of denial.

TABLE 2.1. Symptoms of Panic Attack

A discrete period of intense fear or discomfort, in which four (or more) of the following symptoms develop abruptly and reach a peak within 10 min
1. Palpitations, pounding heart, or accelerated heart rate
2. Sweating
3. Trembling or shaking
4. Sensations of shortness of breath or smothering
5. Feeling of choking
6. Chest pain or discomfort
7. Nausea/abdominal distress
8. Feeling dizzy, lightheaded, or faint
9. Derealization (feelings of unreality) or depersonalization (being detached from oneself)
10. Fear of losing control or going crazy
11. Fear of dying

The patient often will attribute the pain to indigestion or some other insignificant noncardiac problem. It is sometimes hard to believe that, despite crushing chest pain, the onset of the first acute cardiac symptoms can be denied. On the other hand, chest pain, palpitations, and irregular or rapid heartbeats are some of the most common symptoms of many psychiatric disorders.

Of course, just about every patient having chest pain, even if not a classical angina pattern, should at least have an electrocardiogram (ECG). Even when this shows a normal finding, most physicians will consider doing a more extensive cardiac workup, if the symptoms that suggest cardiac disease are recurrent. The tip-off that you may be dealing with a panic disorder include derealization (feelings of unreality), depersonalization (feeling detached from oneself), fear of losing control or going crazy, or an intense fear that one is dying. Sometimes a person with heart disease can have a panic disorder and vice versa. The success rate for treatment of panic disorder where there is a complete remission and the ability to have a normal life is 80% to 90%. This far exceeds the successful treatment of heart disease (Table 2.1).

Another psychiatric disorder that presents with chest pain or other symptoms that overlap with cardiac disease is hypochondriasis. In this situation, the patient misinterprets bodily sensations as symptoms of a serious disease (in this case, cardiac disease). The patient becomes preoccupied with fears that he or she has such a disease. This preoccupation persists, despite appropriate medical evaluation that does not identify cardiac disease and the reassurance of the physician. Frequently, the patient does not recognize that his or her concerns are excessive and unreasonable.

Depression and the Heart

Understanding the relationship between heart disease and depression may not be immediately helpful when called to do a psychiatric consultation on a patient. But, by appreciating this important relationship, you may be able to make more informed decisions about diagnosing depression and making a determination about when and how to treat individual patients. Several dramatic and powerful facts about the connection between depression and heart disease can be very useful to commit to memory (Table 2.2). We often use these pearls in making presentations to cardiologists and in discussions with patients. In our experience, patients who

TABLE 2.2. Clinical Pearls: The Connection between Depression and Cardiac Disease

---

Patients with a history of recurrent depression have a four to five times increased mortality rate at 6-month follow-up after a myocardial infarction (MI) than those without depression

Depression is an independent risk factor for coronary artery disease in both men and women when other cardiovascular risk factors are controlled

Premorbid depression is associated with poor outcome in patients who had postcoronary artery bypass graft; this includes congestive heart failure, mortality, prolonged pain, and failure to return to routine activities

Depression after an MI was associated with increased risk of reinfarction and death

Depression may cause sudden death through the action of the vagus nerve, which causes heart rate variability

Decreased serotonin associated with depression appears to cause changes in platelet stickiness

---

learn this information are more likely to accept referral for psychiatric care.

Type A Personality

One of the most impressive clinical observations made in regard to risk factors is the association of type A personality with CAD (Table 2.3). In some studies, the incidence of CAD in men was twice as high in type A versus non–type A personalities. There is also a positive correlation between type A personality, CAD, and women. Research in this area suggests that type A personality is an independent risk factor

TABLE 2.3. Type A Personality

Hostility
Time urgency
Impatience
Aggressiveness
Competitiveness

(From Friedman M, Rosenman RH. Type A behavior pattern: its association with coronary heart disease. *Ann Clin Res (Finland)* 1971;3(6):300–312.)

for CAD, similar to smoking and hypertension. More recently, a hostility syndrome has been identified, which suggests that anger and aggression are the key factors (Table 2.3).

Social Support

It also has been shown that poor social support can put a person at risk for CAD and increase the death rate from all causes. A patient with CAD who lives alone has a threefold increase in mortality, compared to a patient with a spouse or partner. It may be that those people who are able to relate well to people in their environment will best be able to get help when they need it. Of course, there may be some other pathways that are physiologically based, which will improve the survival of those who are attached.

CASE EXAMPLE: THOSE WHO RELATE WELL WILL BETTER SURVIVE

One of us recalls a grand rounds presentation many years ago by internist Dr. William Green from the University of Rochester Medical School. He told of a research project that he did many years previously when cardiac catheterization had just been instituted. He interviewed patients before and during this procedure and made detailed observations of the patient and recorded information about them. He then subsequently compared his data and other known risk factors with the survival rates of these patients. To the surprise of many, the best predictor of survival was not cardiac function, family history of heart disease, smoking history, or obesity. Instead, the patients who survived the longest were those who related best to Dr. Green during the procedure.

Psychiatric Comorbidity and Lifestyle Risk Factors for Heart Disease

If we look at the classical risk factors for heart disease, excluding depression, which we will discuss later, we can see that each one of them is clearly linked to one or more comorbid psychiatric conditions (Table 2.4).

There is an increasing number of multifaceted programs, such as Dean Ornish's *Program for Reversing Heart Disease* (Ballantine Books, 1992), which address comprehensive

TABLE 2.4. Lifestyle Risk Factors and Comorbid
Psychiatric Conditions

A. Lifestyle risk factors
Overweight
Poor eating habits
Lack of exercise
Substance abuse
Alcohol and drugs
Smoking
**B. Comorbid psychiatric conditions (each can have
   multiple connections to A)**
Personality disorders
Mood disorders
Eating disorders
Alcohol dependency
Drug dependency
Tobacco habituation

---

lifestyle changes, including diet (usually low fat), exercise, stress management training, yoga, meditation, and group therapy. Follow-up research has suggested that overall adherence to such treatment programs are the best predictors of atherosclerotic regression.

PSYCHOLOGICAL ISSUES IN PATIENTS HOSPITALIZED WITH CARDIAC DISEASE

The Intensive Care Unit

Most patients who are suspected of having a myocardial infarction (MI) or patients with acute cardiac failure are admitted to a cardiac care unit (CCU) or another type of intensive care unit (ICU) where they will be monitored and followed up very closely. The initial reaction of most patients to an acute cardiac event and admission to an ICU setting is anxiety and fear. The defense mechanism, denial, has usually been breached by this point. Some patients will manifest extreme anxiety, terror, and panic. On some level, there will be death anxiety, as most people associate an ICU with life-threatening situations. As the cardiac symptoms (i.e., chest pain and shortness of breath) subside, there may be a lessening of the anxiety. In addition, morphine sulfate, which is often given to patients with cardiac pain, will cause both sedation and relaxation.

Cardiac monitoring equipment often reassures patients, as they feel that they are being closely watched and that any abnormality can be dealt with immediately. On the other hand, if patients who are hooked up to a monitor are not informed about what to expect, they can be made more anxious by observing a movement artifact on their ECG monitor or by misinterpreting various beeps and alarms. While it should be the role of the cardiac team to explain these things to the patient, sometimes this task falls to the psychiatric consultant.

You will see a wide range of behaviors under these circumstances, which can be accounted for by the patient's personality and psychiatric makeup. It is not unusual, for example, to see patients who insist on signing out of the CCU or ICU because they cannot tolerate their anxiety in this setting. They may experience the forced confinement as a threat to their sense of control. Listening to these patients and trying to address, reassure, or interpret their concerns can be helpful, as can recommending medication, as indicated later in this chapter. Other patients will regress, becoming whiney and dependent. Both these extremes can be very provocative to the medical and nursing staff, especially to those who have not had a great deal of experience in these settings. Brief supportive discussion with staff in this situation can be very helpful.

Open Heart Surgery

See Chapter 11 on surgery. Patients undergoing cardiac surgery will of course often spend time postoperatively in the ICU as described earlier.

Left Ventricular Assist Devices

Left ventricular assist devices (LVADs) are used to reverse end-organ dysfunction and sustain life for patients who are awaiting transplants. These devices can be used at home and in the hospital. Patients who are given these devices are often severely medically compromised and can develop a delirium that needs to be treated, depending on the etiology. Depression is often present, and patients should be evaluated and treated accordingly.

Defibrillators

Modern technology has developed a device that can automatically and successfully defibrillate the patient who would otherwise experience sudden death due to ventricular tachycardia and ventricular fibrillation. These devices may be worn externally or implanted under the skin. The devices can read the ECG and deliver a shock that will cardiovert the heart to normal rhythm. The patient may or may not lose consciousness before receiving the cardioversion. The shocks may be experienced as a painful blow to the chest and may be repeated several times in succession. As you might imagine, patients who undergo this experience can develop marked anticipatory anxiety, phobias, as well as a chronic anxiety state. They may develop symptoms of posttraumatic stress disorder (PTSD), not unlike people who have experienced repeated electrical shocks. We suggest a creative therapeutic approach that may include medication and various types of individual or group therapy. There are self-help groups available for patients with defibrillators and their families and you should refer patients to these if possible.

Pacemakers

To a lesser degree, patients with implanted pacemakers may have psychological reactions. However, because the patient rarely has any awareness of the operation of this device, it is easier for him or her to adjust to it. Pacemaker technology has improved dramatically. It is now more efficient, effective, and safe and there can be no restriction to lifestyle.

TREATMENT ISSUES

Treatment of Acute Anxiety and Fear in the Cardiac Patient

Psychotherapeutic Approaches

Quiet reassurance is usually the first-line treatment for fear and anxiety with heart disease or any other condition. Begin by listening to the patient. Does the patient have a "nemesis complex" in which he or she expects to get sick and possibly die of heart disease in the same way and at the same age as a close relative? Has someone close to him or her had similar symptoms and, if so, what happened to that person? Does the patient have multiple people with cardiac disease in his or her family? Does your patient understand the typical healing process from a cardiac procedure and that in many cases he or she will be expected to return to normal activities in several weeks? If the prognosis is grave, is your patient reassured that pain will be controlled and (if true) that there is a chance for cardiac surgery and perhaps cardiac transplant?

When a patient utilizes denial, he or she is usually defending against anxiety, fear, and depression. On some level, the patient is afraid that these feelings will be overwhelming. The patient who is scared, even paranoid, and wants to sign out should be approached in a nonconfrontational manner. Such patients need to hear that their condition is treatable, but that they need to be in the hospital at this time. This can be reinforced by hearing the same message from trusted family members and from their outside physician, by phone, if necessary. In most cases, the patient can be persuaded to continue inpatient treatment. In our experience, it is rare that such a patient would meet criteria for an involuntary psychiatric admission.

Medications

Benzodiazepines

Fear and anxiety can be treated by medication. In cases of an acute MI, even when the patient is outwardly calm, it is reasonable to be concerned that any hidden anxiety may lead to an autonomic instability that can endanger the patient's life at this time. Therefore, in most cases in the CCU, benzodiazepines are the first line of medication. The choice of a benzodiazepine usually depends on the rapidity of action that is desired, routes available, and the preference of long- or short-acting benzodiazepine. All medications can do the job if properly used, and the experience of the physician often determines the choice. For rapid tranquilization, we prefer lorazepam, alprazolam, clorazepate, or diazepam. The latter is longer acting, with the half-life varying between 20 and 60 hours and saturation occurring after 2 or 3 days. Although some patients may prefer to take a tranquilizer every 3 or 4 hours immediately after the cardiac incident, we prefer, when feasible, to switch the patient to clonazepam, which achieves maximum concentration in 1 to 4 hours, and the half-life is typically 30 to 40 hours. We have found that often this can be given once or twice per day and it gives an even tranquilizing effect for at least 15 hours. Sedation is a potential side effect of all benzodiazepines and it can be synergistic for this effect with other medications that sedate, particularly with morphine or other narcotics. Other benzodiazepines have been specifically used for sleep medications, and any medication in this class can facilitate sleep. Oversedation is usually not desired, as it can reduce respiration and make the patient susceptible to aspiration pneumonia. In the ICU and CCU, patients are closely monitored so oversedation is highly unlikely to occur.

The patient's age and medical condition must always be taken into consideration in choosing a benzodiazepine. Accumulation of this class of drugs can occur in geriatric patients and/or patients with liver damage. "Start low and go slow" is always the rule of thumb in these situations. There also can be a possible rare paradoxical effect with a potential rage response when patients are given this class of drugs. Parenteral forms of chlordiazepoxide and diazepam are available, although intramuscular (IM) absorption is not very predictable. Cautious intravenous (IV) administration of these drugs or lorazepam is used in situations where oral administration is not feasible.

The sustained use of benzodiazepines can cause tolerance and physical dependence. Patients who were on benzodiazepines before the cardiac event that brought them to the hospital should be continued on such medication or withdrawal symptoms, including fatal seizures, can occur. The benzodiazepines can be tapered and withdrawn, if clinically indicated.

Neuroleptics

In cases where there is psychotic manifestation or there has been severe anxiety that has been difficult to control, we suggest the use of neuroleptics. This is also the case and may be the drug of choice when there is a delirium. Delirium is more common in postoperative patients after cardiac surgery. Low-dosage haloperidol is usually the drug of first choice in this setting and can be administered orally or parenterally. Before IV haloperidol is administered, the IV line should be flushed with 2 mL of normal saline. The IV bolus initial dosage of haloperidol is usually 0.5 mg, but it can be increased to as high as 10 to 20 mg. Sometimes it can be alternated with 1 mg IV of lorazepam given to patients at 30-minute intervals between medications while the patient is closely monitored. The atypical neuroleptics may prove to have a role here. The treatment of delirium is discussed in more detail in Chapter 10.

Treatment of Depression in the Cardiac Patient

Antidepressants

Usually it is not necessary to initiate antidepressant medication to patients in the CCU or ICU. Depressive symptoms first seen here usually are related to acute adjustment problems or to the beginning of an acute grieving response that is related to anticipated losses. Before starting antidepressants, it is most often advisable to first sort out these situations over several visits that generally continue after release from the intensive care setting and sometimes after release from the hospital. Because it takes at least a few weeks to achieve the therapeutic effect of such medication, the consultant should not feel under pressure to institute this medication, unless there is a clear indication.

You may be questioned about continuing antidepressant medication that the patient was taking before the cardiac event. In most cases, if the patient is taking pills and liquids by mouth, it is usually a good idea to continue such medication, especially if there is a likelihood of a discontinuation syndrome, such as that which occurs frequently with shorter-acting selective serotonin reuptake inhibitors (SSRIs), such as paroxetine. An exception might be in those rare cases where a patient was taking a monoamine oxidase inhibitor (MAOI) that can cause a hypertensive crisis in interaction with some medications often given in the ICU. Other potential drug interactions are discussed later in this chapter.

Mood Stabilizers

As is the case with antidepressants, it is rare that a mood stabilizer will need to be introduced to a patient who is receiving intensive care. Such decisions usually are made at a later date. Agitated behavior usually is dealt with by the use of benzodiazepines and/or neuroleptics. In rare cases where true manic behavior is diagnosed in a bipolar patient in the ICU, the usual treatment of mania with lithium, valproate, or another mood stabilizer could be started.

Psychiatrists frequently are consulted when a patient who is already on a mood stabilizer is admitted to the ICU after an acute event, such as a heart attack. Our usual approach in these situations is to hold off on continuing lithium, especially because there are invariably abrupt changes in diet or the patient could be made NPO and IV therapy might be run. Patients are more likely to become lithium toxic in such situations. It is unlikely that an acute manic attack would suddenly develop within a few days of being off lithium (and, if one did occur, it could be easily treated).

Psychiatric Effects of Drugs Used to Treat Cardiovascular Disease

This abbreviated list will give the reader some idea of the potential psychiatric effects of some of the medications commonly used to treat cardiovascular conditions.

- Antiarrhythmics (e.g., procainamide, flecainide, disopyramide, mexiletine)—effects include depression and confusion.
- Beta-blockers (e.g., propranolol)—depression is a frequent effect. Less common side effects are vivid dreams, nightmares, and even psychotic manifestations. The newer beta-blockers, such as atenolol and metoprolol, are more cardioselective and may have fewer psychiatric effects.
- Antihypertensives
   Reserpine (has fallen into disuse, but is still a component of some combination drugs still in the market)—depression may occur.
   Methyldopa—depression, impaired concentration, hallucinations, paranoia, and other psychotic manifestations may occur.
   Clonidine—effects are similar to above, but are less severe.
   Calcium channel blockers (e.g., verapamil, nifedipine and diltiazem, nimodipine, and amlodipine)—effects are depression and confusion.
   Prazosin—increased anxiety and depression can occur.
   Angiotensin-converting enzyme (ACE) inhibitors (e.g., captopril, enalapril, quinapril, and ramipril)—effects include nervousness, depression, and decreased libido.
- Digitalis preparations—effects include depression, hallucinations, and delirium.

Cardiovascular Effects of Drugs Used to Treat Psychiatric Conditions

This list is also far from complete. It also should be appreciated that when there are effects, they are much more likely to occur in patients who have preexisting cardiovascular pathology.

- SSRIs—The psychiatric drugs in this important category do not routinely cause cardiovascular side effects, even in patients with preexisting cardiovascular disease. However, isolated reports have given examples of arrhythmias and vasoconstriction of damaged vessels that were believed to have been related to the use of the medication.

- Tricyclic antidepressants (TCAs)—Cardiovascular side effects have made this group mostly a backup group of antidepressants, once SSRIs were proved to be effective. TCAs can cause orthostatic hypotension and conduction defects, such as increased PR, QRS, and QT intervals with potential primary, secondary, and tertiary heart block. TCAs also can cause sinus tachycardia, supraventricular tachyarrhythmias, ventricular tachycardia, and ventricular fibrillation. Severe cardiac effects are common with overdoses.

- Other antidepressants

  Venlafaxine—This medication blocks neuronal uptake of serotonin and norepinephrine and can cause some elevation of blood pressure, particularly in high dosages. Therefore, blood pressure should be monitored when administering this medication.

  Bupropion—This monocyclic antidepressant is presumed to inhibit dopamine reuptake. It is shown to cause occasional postural hypotension or even hypertension. It has been shown to foster smoking cessation and therefore is potentially helpful in the treatment plan of patients with cardiovascular disease.

  Trazodone—Some consider this medication to be a newer version of the tricyclics. It has been very popular as an adjunctive medication with the SSRIs to assist with sleep. It has less cardiovascular effects than the older TCAs, but it can cause postural hypotension and many types of arrhythmias. Particular caution should be paid if given with medications known to cause QT prolongation.

- MAOIs—There is the potential for serious hypertensive crisis with this medication, if foods such as those rich in tyramine are not avoided. This also can occur in interaction with certain cold medicines, many other antidepressants, and meperidine. A common side effect is postural hypotension.

- Methylphenidate and other stimulants—Methylphenidate is contraindicated for patients with hypertension. Blood pressure should be monitored closely in patients taking this drug. Acute overdose of methylphenidate and other stimulants can lead to serious cardiovascular symptoms, such as labile blood pressure, cardiac arrhythmias, and circulatory collapse.

- Mood stabilizers—Lithium can cause minor ST-T wave changes in the ECG. However, in cases of lithium toxicity there may be conduction disturbances and arrhythmias.
- Neuroleptics—There has been renewed interest in the fact that certain neuroleptics increase QT intervals, which may result in a variety of symptoms from syncope and palpitations to tachyarrhythmias and sudden death. In a study of commonly used neuroleptics, thioridazine was most associated with a higher percentage of patients with prolonged QT, followed by ziprasidone, quetiapine, risperidone, haloperidol, and olanzapine. In addition, another cardiovascular effect of neuroleptics is hypotension. Clozapine, chlorpromazine, thioridazine, and mesoridazine are most likely to produce significant hypotension. Haloperidol is the least likely to produce hypotension.

Drug Interactions

Although it may seem a daunting task, as a consultant, it is your responsibility to be familiar with all possible drug–drug interactions of any medication that you are recommending or reviewing. The Physicians' Desk Reference (PDR), hospital databases, and new software programs will be helpful. Although there are dozens, if not hundreds, of theoretical drug–drug interactions, in reality, there are relatively few clinically significant ones. In general, drug interactions are not contraindications, but they require increased monitoring. Listed in the subsequent text are some important drug interactions between psychotropic drugs and medications that are used in treatment of cardiac disease.

- SSRIs—High protein binding affinity can affect levels of digoxin. One study has shown increased level of digoxin when given with paroxetine. Another study documented an increased prothrombin time when fluoxetine and warfarin were combined. Prothrombin time should be closely monitored whenever any SSRI and warfarin are given together.
- Phenothiazines—When ACE inhibitors are given with phenothiazine, particularly the low potency ones (e.g., chlorpromazine), there can be significant hypotension and orthostasis.

- Benzodiazepines—If benzodiazepines are combined with calcium channel blockers, such as diltiazem and verapamil, the benzodiazepine level may be increased with increased sedative effect. Cholestyramine can reduce the levels of lorazepam. Benzodiazepines can increase serum digoxin levels.
- Carbamazepine and lithium—Calcium channel blockers can increase levels of both lithium and carbamazepine. Lithium levels can change abruptly when a diuretic is given; therefore, the patient should be monitored closely under these circumstances. ACE inhibitors can increase lithium retention, and beta-blockers may reduce the renal clearance of lithium as well.
- Valproate—Cholestyramine reduces absorption of valproate.

OTHER ISSUES IN PSYCHOCARDIOLOGY

Sex and Heart Disease

Any extreme physical or emotional exertion can precipitate angina or an MI in a patient with significant heart disease. This could theoretically include sexual activity, although it is rarely the case. Anecdotal stories of sudden death due to a cardiac event that occurs during sexual liaisons will sometimes cause cardiac patients to avoid sex altogether. Such concerns are particularly common among patients and their spouses in the immediate postdischarge period following a heart attack. Most cardiologists feel that patients can resume sexual activity, provided they do not have angina. In the presence of angina, patients may be advised to take nitroglycerine medication before engaging in sexual activity, much as they would be advised to do before walking up a flight of stairs. There is often embarrassment, shame, and guilt on the part of the patient and partner about this topic. You may need to explore this topic with the couple while the patient is in the hospital, and a referral for short-term psychotherapy may be helpful, if there are conflict and difficulties in this area.

The use of anti-impotence medications, such as sildenafil (Viagra) and other similar medications, have opened a new dimension for the treatment of erectile dysfunction. It is important to recognize that these medications are contraindicated in patients who are taking nitrates for the treatment of cardiac conditions. Even patients with significant CAD who are not taking nitrates should be cautioned about them because the medication can improve sexual activity so quickly that the patient may overdo it, putting dangerous strain on his or her cardiac reserve.

LIAISON POTENTIAL

In view of the mounting evidence that connects depression and heart disease, it makes sense for a consultation-liaison (C-L) psychiatrist to work closely with cardiologists and cardiology programs. In cases where there is a comprehensive program that includes preventative care, psychiatrists may be able to offer unique skills in the development of special programs, as well as in providing direct services. Some examples of liaison work that a C-L psychiatrist can do in the area of psychocardiology include the following:

1. Run stress reduction groups.
2. Participate in planning and running programs that address lifestyle changes.
3. Conduct regular rounds in the CCU, see patients, and meet with staff.
4. Become a member of the transplant team.
5. Speak regularly to the heart club of cardiac patients and their families.
6. Occasionally speak to special groups of transplant or defibrillator patients and their families.
7. Participate in smoking cessation programs.

3

Psychooncology

Essential Concepts
- Many people incorrectly view any diagnosis of cancer as an automatic "death sentence."
- This misconception contributes to cancer phobia in people who might not have cancer and to the pathological use of denial in people who may have symptoms of cancer.
- Most people who have had a close relative with cancer develop a "nemesis complex" in which they fear getting that cancer at a similar age.
- More than 50% of cancer patients have at least one of these three psychiatric disorders: adjustment disorder, anxiety disorder, or depressive disorder.
- Never accept a cancer patient's depressive symptoms as "par for the course." Instead, treat these symptoms aggressively, using the full range of available psychopharmacologic and therapeutic techniques.

It used to be that if you were asked to consult on a patient with cancer, it meant that you were being asked to help the patient cope with the process of dying. Commonly, patients with cancer experience fears of disfigurement, disability, dependence, and dying a painful death. This is no longer the case. Treatments for cancer have become more effective and sophisticated. Patients survive for much longer, and you should become familiar with a range of complex psychological issues that are frequently brought up by patients who are facing this illness. Many modern cancer centers have a team of mental health professionals who address the stress of patients and family members, provide psychosocial education, and enhance the development of therapeutic communication skills for the oncology staff.

THE DIAGNOSIS OF CANCER

Cancer Phobia

Many people have a tremendous fear of cancer, which can dominate their lives. This fear often stems from the fact that 25 to 50 years ago most cancers could not be effectively treated and people tended to view the diagnosis of cancer as "an automatic death sentence." Although great strides have been made in early diagnosis and treatment, many people still view the cancer label with a similar dread. This should be foremost in your mind when speaking with a patient who may be faced with a cancer diagnosis. When you encounter such patients, you should look for what is known as the *nemesis complex*, in which the patient expects to be struck down with the same illness as the parents or other relatives at a specific age. Also, when dealing with a patient with a cancer phobia, the clinician should look for other conflicts with which the patient may be struggling, as illustrated in the following case.

CASE VIGNETTE: "NOT LIKE MY MOTHER"

The patient is a 69-year-old retired schoolteacher, mother of four grown children, and married for 40 years to "my best friend." She had no previous psychiatric history and had shown very good adjustment through a life-threatening motor vehicle accident 5 years previously, which required hospitalization for 2 months. The patient was now status post simple mastectomy for breast cancer and was undergoing follow-up chemotherapy. On the basis of her circumscribed lesion and the absence of lymph nodes or metastasis, her prognosis was considered to be quite good.

However, the patient was noted to be extremely anxious and fearful. She was sleeping poorly, both during a brief hospitalization for chemotherapy and at home. She became obsessed with having a discussion of her living will with each of her children and was particularly concerned that her husband would not honor her wishes for no heroic care, should that be necessary.

The patient agreed to meet with the consultation-liaison (C-L) psychiatrist whom she had seen as part of her routine care during recovery from the motor vehicle injury. She shared her deep concern and recurrent dreams that she would die in agonizing pain. She had cared for her mother who had ovarian cancer at the age of 68 and who had died of metastatic disease after 6 months of hospitalization. She believed that the doctors had been afraid of "addicting" her mother to pain medication for much of this time. Her brother had insisted on experimental treatment during the later stages of treatment. The patient was with her mother daily and has lived with the memories of her pleas to end her life, which she did not know how to grant. She has lived with the expectation that she would get cancer when she reached the age at which her mother became ill.

With the patient's permission, the psychiatrist was able to hold a series of meetings with the patient, doctors, and family. The patient was reassured that her prognosis was good, but that the doctors were advocates of palliative care, which included good pain control, should that be needed. The doctors and family also reviewed the patient's wishes that no heroic methods would be taken if her condition were to become terminal. The open discussion brought the patient and the family closer together.

Psychological Responses to the Diagnosis of Cancer

There are several stages that patients often go through before they can accept a diagnosis of cancer. These are similar to the stages in the dying patient that were originally described by Kubler-Ross. Rather than marching through these stages in a stepwise manner, real patients move back and forth between the stages. Understanding the dynamics of each stage will help the consultant navigate many of the psychological complications in working with a patient who is newly diagnosed with cancer.

- **Denial**—The extreme example of denial would be a woman who first presents to a physician with a fungating breast mass or a patient who has lost a large amount of weight before seeking medical attention. Another example would be a man with bloody stools for 1 year who has been weak and tired and who has had loss of appetite. You should be alert to the possibility that the patient with marked denial may be delusional or have an extremely fragile ego. When finally confronted with the reality of their illness and its treatment, such patients may become suicidal. Other forms of denial are more subtle and have to do with patients being overly optimistic and not considering the possibility of a serious prognosis. Remember that some degree of denial can be adaptive, especially if it is not interfering with your patient receiving adequate treatment.

- **Anger**—Psychiatrists are frequently called when patients are angry and hostile toward their doctors and the treatment team. This may be manifested by the patient refusing diagnostic tests, wishing to change doctors, or requesting to sign out of the hospital against medical advice. This could be a defensive response to the new diagnosis of cancer. During this stage, the patient can show very provocative behavior, which can be directed toward the consulting psychiatrist or the medical–surgical treating team. You should be prepared to help your medical colleagues understand and deal with these reactions. Chapter 16 presents a full discussion of such psychotherapeutic techniques.

- **Bargaining**—In this stage, patients will bargain with God or fate, promising to live a better, moral, or different life if they should survive this illness. It is at this point that patients may overidealize their oncologists and become quite attached or dependent on them. They assume that the doctor has the power to make their bargained wish come true. If the patient's treatment goes poorly, the doctor could be blamed and this could lead to a disruption of the doctor–patient relationship.

- **Acceptance**—This could mean different things to different people. A patient may accept the diagnosis of cancer, but may not yet be ready to accept the serious prognosis. Another patient may have passed through all the stages outlined earlier and may have accepted the fact that he or she is in the terminal phase of life. Acceptance of the diagnosis of cancer allows patients to explore all treatment options, as well as mobilize support systems. It allows them to regain a sense of control over their illness so that they can now go on with the process of living their lives, even while they are dying.

ANXIETY AND CANCER

Anxiety is a common reaction to cancer, and we recommend that you explore the specific origins of your patient's fears.

The most common causes of anxiety among cancer patients include the following:

1. Fear of the unknown creates a sense of free-floating anxiety.
2. Fear of death creates anxiety that is related to separation anxiety (i.e., fear of separation from loved ones and memories of separations from parents).
3. Fear of mutilation creates anxiety that is related to universal fears of damage to body integrity, sexual organs or function, and distortion of body image.
4. Fear of closed spaces (claustrophobia) creates anxiety that can be activated by having magnetic resonance imaging (MRI) or other procedures in closed spaces, prolonged hospitalizations, being confined to bed, or underlying fantasies about dying and being in a coffin.
5. Fear of recurrent physical symptoms creates anxiety, such as anticipation of pain or nausea and vomiting from chemotherapy or from the illness itself.

Table 3.1 presents an overview of the different types of anxiety related to cancer.

Anxiety is best treated by establishing an empathic supportive relationship in which your patient feels safe enough with you to ventilate and explore concerns, fantasies, and misconceptions about his or her illness. Use cognitive therapy strategies to correct erroneous beliefs about cancer and teach your patient stress reduction and relaxation techniques.

Adjunctive use of psychopharmacology also can be quite helpful. Become familiar with the use of antianxiety medications, such as benzodiazepines and buspirone, as well as atypical and typical neuroleptics. Selective serotonin reuptake inhibitors (SSRIs) are also quite effective for panic and anxiety symptoms in cancer patients.

DEPRESSION AND CANCER

It is estimated that one fourth to one third of patients with cancer have unrecognized and untreated depression. The risk is even higher in hospitalized patients and patients with more advanced disease. Symptoms include insomnia, poor appetite, anhedonia, anergia, anxiety, irritability, impaired concentration, and suicidality. The diagnosis is often missed because the clinician believes that these symptoms are the result of the physical illness itself. At times, patients' families,

TABLE 3.1. Causes of Anxiety in Patients with Cancer

Situational
Diagnosis of cancer, prognosis discussion
Crisis, illness/treatment
Conflicts with family or staff
Anticipating a frightening procedure
Awaiting results of tests
Fears of recurrence following completion of treatment
Disease related
Poorly controlled pain
Abnormal metabolic states
Hormone-secreting tumors
Paraneoplastic syndromes (remote central nervous system effects)
Treatment related
Frightening or painful procedures (magnetic resonance imaging, scans, wound debridement)
Anxiety-producing drugs (antiemetic neuroleptics, bronchodilators)
Withdrawal states (opioids, benzodiazepines, alcohol)
Conditioned (anticipatory) anxiety, nausea, and vomiting with cyclic chemotherapy
Exacerbation of preexisting anxiety disorder
Phobias (needles, claustrophobia)
Panic or generalized anxiety disorder
Posttraumatic stress disorder (Holocaust survivors, Vietnam veterans, recall of the death of a relative with cancer)
Obsessive compulsive disorder

(Reprinted with permission from Holland JC, Friedlander M. Oncology. In: Blumenfield M, Strain JJ, eds. *Psychosomatic medicine*. Philadelphia: Lippincott Williams & Wilkins, 2006:132.)

and even clinicians, feel that depression is expected or "par for the course" in patients who have a diagnosis of cancer.

The diagnosis of depression in a cancer patient can be made when depressive symptoms persist for at least 2 weeks and when cognitive symptoms, such as low self-esteem, hopelessness, helplessness, self-deprecation, and varying degrees of suicidality, are prominent.

The relationship between depression and cancer is complex. Clearly, cancer can trigger a major depression. Some of the medications and other medically related risk factors for depression in the cancer patient are noted in the Table 3.2.

TABLE 3.2. Medical-Related Risk Factors for Depression in Patients with Cancer

---

Poorly controlled pain
Other chronic disease/disability; advanced stage
Medications
  Corticosteroids
    Prednisone, dexamethasone
  Interferon and interleukin-2
  Chemotherapeutic agents
    Vincristine, vinblastine, procarbazine, L-asparaginase
Other medications
  Cimetidine
  Indomethacin
  Levodopa
  Methyldopa
  Pentazocine
  Phenmetrazine
  Phenobarbital
  Propranolol
  Rauwolfia alkaloids
  Tamoxifen
  Antibiotics
  Amphotericin B
Other medical conditions
  Metabolic (anemia, hypercalcemia)
  Nutritional (vitamin B_{12} or folate deficiency)
  Endocrine (hyperthyroidism or hypothyroidism, adrenal
    insufficiency)
  Neurologic (paraneoplastic syndromes)
Sites of cancer
  Pancreatic, small cell lung, breast cancer, lymphoma
    (producing remote central nervous system effects)

(Reprinted with permission from Holland JC, Friedlander M. Oncology. In: Blumenfield M, Strain JJ, eds. *Psychosomatic medicine*. Philadelphia: Lippincott Williams & Wilkins, 2006:134.)

There are some suggestions in the research literature that mood states can trigger or aggravate the course of cancer. There have been reports that breast cancer patients who have a "fighting spirit" have a higher survival rate than those who stoically accept their illness. In addition, there is an increased cancer mortality rate in widows, compared to never-married or married women.

Although these findings are suggestive, there has been no substantial evidence in the literature proving that depression can actually cause cancer. Obviously, we would strongly discourage you from implying to your patients that they have somehow caused their illness because this is probably always false and is certainly demoralizing.

Treatment of Depression in the Cancer Patient

Depression in cancer patients is best managed utilizing a combination of supportive psychotherapy, cognitive behavioral therapy (CBT), and psychopharmacology.

Medication Treatment

Because patients with cancer often are debilitated and have other medical complications, we recommend that you "start low, go slow." It is important to remember that these patients are usually on a lot of different medications. It is advisable to look up drug interactions before prescribing any medication. The use of these medications is reviewed in Chapter 2. SSRIs, in particular, have a good track record in cancer patients.

Sometimes patients with cancer can become acutely depressed with a cessation or near-cessation of nutritional intake, marked reduction in psychomotor activity, and minimal communication. You may not be sure if this is a depressive state or a progressive deterioration of their medical condition. The patient could very well respond to standard antidepressant therapy eventually, but if the depression is life threatening, you do not have the luxury of waiting several weeks. In this situation, we often try psychostimulants. You can start with dextroamphetamine (2.5 mg in the morning and at noon), gradually titrating the dose upward from there. If the patient is going to respond at all, it is usually immediate, and you will very rapidly note improved intake and communication. This stimulant can be continued for up to several weeks, while the standard antidepressant is being instituted. If the symptoms recur, it can be restarted and, if necessary, continued on a long-term basis.

As with any psychostimulant, remember to exercise caution if your patient is prone to develop hypertension, and we recommend a cardiology consultation for patients with cardiac disease. Methylphenidate can also be used as a stimulant.

CASE VIGNETTE: "THE FIREMAN WHO NEEDED A JUMP START"

A 72-year-old retired fireman with lung cancer was status post partial lung resection and had recently completed a cycle of chemotherapy. He had stopped eating abruptly and appeared to have given up. The patient had a history of heavy drinking, but had not been drinking for the previous 5 years. His family noted that he had been withdrawn and depressed for approximately 6 months after his wife died, but he seemed to be recovering at the time that he developed pneumonia and cancer was diagnosed.

When seen by the C-L psychiatrist, he seemed quite distracted. It was difficult to tell if he was oriented, but, after much effort, it was clear that he knew where he was and what year it was. His affect was bland and he denied being very depressed or suicidal. He did not cooperate for a complete mental status examination. Neurologic examination as well as MRI of the head were within normal limits although the consultant did raise the question of whether the patient had developed metastasis to the brain that was not yet detected. Delirium was considered, but was not substantiated by other components of the mental status examination.

The decision was made to put the patient on fluoxetine, initially 10 mg and then raising it 20 mg per day within 4 days. However, there was concern that the patient's condition was deteriorating and that any antidepressant effect might take several weeks. The patient's cardiac status and blood pressure were stable, and it was decided to put the patient on methylphenidate (5 mg in the morning). Improvement was noted almost immediately, and the patient began to speak more freely and began to eat. After 5 days, there was a return to previous symptoms. The dosage was then titrated up to 15 mg per day over the next 5 days. The patient showed marked improvement and gained several pounds over the next 2 weeks. He began to converse and laugh with his family. The psychostimulant was discontinued after 2 weeks and the fluoxetine was titrated to 40 mg per day. The patient continued to do well and was discharged from the hospital for outpatient medical and psychiatric follow-up.

Psychotherapeutic Issues

Medical surgical effects of a particular cancer and treatment—Although it may seem obvious, it is important to remember that cancer and its treatment profoundly and negatively affect the victim's body. After cancer treatment, your patient may find himself or herself unable to walk, talk, eat, or breathe without special assistance. Other common symptoms include persistent weakness, fatigue, nausea, and vomiting. Severe weight loss often occurs as a direct effect of cancer, while both weight gain and hair loss can result from chemotherapy.

All of these physical changes typically affect a patient's self and body image and can contribute to profound depression. There may be a grieving process for the loss (or the anticipated loss) of a body part or body function. As with grieving of interpersonal loss, you may notice that your patient becomes preoccupied with the lost object and its meaning. Your patient will go through episodic relapses of intense feelings as he or she moves toward some kind of acceptance. If your depressed patient has not already brought these issues up, then you should because they are difficult, but very important, issues.

For some patients, the inability to function sexually, to have children, or to be considered a sexual being can be devastating, whether this is brought about by disfigurement or loss of function. Although these issues are especially relevant in patients with cancer of the breast, uterus, prostate, and testis, many other types of cancer have the potential for similar impact through systemic effects, indirect anatomic involvement, and by the nature of the surgery, chemotherapy, or radiation used for treatment.

Environmental factors—Research has shown that patients with fewer social supports generally have a poorer prognosis and develop poorer coping skills in response to their illness. Therefore, you should encourage your patient to reach out to friends and family members and reinforce the involvement of supportive people when you meet with them. Of course, be sensitive to individual situations in which family involvement may be adding fuel to the fire because of long-standing interpersonal conflicts.

A variety of local and national self-help groups are available to your patients; become informed about such organizations in your area and make appropriate referrals. The Internet is becoming increasingly helpful for cancer patients seeking support and education. There is a list of relevant websites and URLs at the end of this book.

Psychological makeup—Carefully assess your patient's character and personality traits because these have great bearing on the ability to adapt positively to serious illness. Optimism, a sense of humor, and the ability to reframe a negative experience into a positive one are helpful traits that should be encouraged. On the other hand, the tendency to worry and to feel pessimistic about one's self-worth and future are broadly defined in the research literature as "neuroticism," and have been associated with poor emotional adjustment.

Nemesis complex—Make sure to assess your patient's family history of cancer. Ask about the course of illness, including recurrences, in persons who were meaningful and important to the patient. If your patient has cared directly for a cancer victim, find out what he or she may have witnessed in terms of pain and suffering because the memory of such experiences will often influence fears and expectations for the patient. When the person cared for has been a parent, there is often a deep-seated expectation that the patient will suffer the same fate. Bringing such ideas out in the open can often give relief and allow for a realistic assessment.

Distorted communication—Over and over again, in our work with cancer patients, we are struck with distortions in communication. Of all illnesses, cancer is the most difficult to discuss because of its unspoken aura of imminent death. It is not unusual for the treating physician to request psychiatric consultation for a patient who has not been informed of the cancer diagnosis. This deception may be perpetuated by the patient's family. On the other hand, we have also encountered patients with cancer who request that the family not be informed of the diagnosis. Even when the diagnosis is out in the open, patients and families may try to conceal from each other the prognosis or the terminal nature of the disease.

We approach such situations by asking the patient and family what they imagine the diagnosis or prognosis will reveal. Often enough, it turns out that those persons who others were trying to deceive actually understood the truth. When this is not the case, a careful analysis of why the true nature of the illness is being withheld will be helpful in determining the best path to follow in these delicate situations. Sometimes both parties feel that they must "protect" the other party. When there are close emotional ties, the anticipated loss is so powerful that both parties find it very difficult to discuss.

In some cases, a patient will ignore communications about the seriousness of the cancer as part of the defense mechanism of denial. Patients use denial when they experience a serious threat to their identity and sense of wholeness. Truth for the sake of truth usually is not the best guiding principle to use here. Defenses are not readily given up, unless there is something of value to replace them. In such situations, you should work to establish a good rapport before beginning to confront the reality of the disease. A good working alliance with the therapist often will sustain a patient as he or she gives up defenses.

PSYCHIATRIC ISSUES RELATED TO SPECIFIC TYPES OF CANCER

Breast cancer—One out of nine women will develop breast cancer in their lifetime. In 2001, breast cancer was estimated to have been newly diagnosed every 3 minutes, and a woman died from breast cancer every 13 minutes. The risk is three times higher for those women who have a first-degree relative with the disease. Women with a strong family history of breast cancer will sometimes choose elective bilateral mastectomy before they show any signs of pathology, especially if they have genetic markers that indicate a high probability of developing cancer. Patients who undergo radical mastectomy often develop a variety of psychological problems that range from a sense of loss and poor self-esteem to significant depression. Breast reconstruction with implants is an option for many and can be quite helpful psychologically. Both individual therapy and group therapy have been shown to be quite effective for breast cancer patients. Research data has suggested that psychotherapeutic efforts will be more effective if instituted during the initial stages of diagnosis and treatment.

Gynecologic cancer—Although regular Pap smears can be lifesaving, a lack of education as well as self-consciousness and shame can sometimes cause women to avoid this important screening test. Treatment of gynecologic cancer often leads to sexual dysfunction. Involvement of the patient's partner in most psychotherapeutic encounters is useful. The loss of fertility after cancer treatment also can be a major psychological blow. Studies have shown that women with gynecologic cancer have a higher rate of depression than similarly aged cohorts.

Prostate cancer—Many of the issues discussed under "gynecologic cancer" apply to men with prostate cancer. Some men refuse a screening rectal examination, either through ignorance of the dangers of prostate cancer or because of a belief that inserting something in their anus will compromise their masculinity. Once diagnosed and treated, both impotence and incontinence are common, leading to issues of embarrassment and shame, which, in turn, can trigger psychiatric syndromes. Support groups have been very helpful for men with such problems.

Hodgkin's disease and cancer of the testes—These cancers can cause infertility, particularly in relatively young men with subsequent emotional difficulties. Preservation of sperm before treatment can be offered as an option to these men. Patients with Hodgkin's disease often have fatigue, depression, anxiety, and irritability during treatment, in addition to infertility. Psychological concerns in survivors often relate to the slow return of their energy levels and the fear of recurrence of disease.

Pancreatic cancer—It is an old clinical pearl that patients with this type of cancer can present with dysphoric mood before any other symptoms of the disease. Various studies have shown evidence that depression and some anxiety were more frequent in patients with pancreatic cancer than in patients with other intra-abdominal tumors. Often these symptoms precede the appearance of physical symptoms of the disease. Several biologic pathways, using neurobiologic, metabolic, and neuroendocrine mechanisms, have been postulated as possible causes.

Brain tumors—Brain tumors can present with changes in mental status, including depression, delirium, dementia, or seizures. Partial complex seizures without motor symptoms also can signal the onset of a tumor. Brain tumors are best diagnosed by brain imaging with contrast. Any patient having a first psychotic break after the age of 40 should have brain imaging to rule out a tumor. Certain cancers are more likely to metastasize to the brain and to present with changes in mental status. Lung cancer is the most common tumor to metastasize to the brain, with 10% of cases at onset and 30% at a later point in the disease, which may be at any time before the patient succumbs to the cancer. At any point in the course of the disease, patients with breast cancer can develop brain metastases in 6% to 20% of cases.

Patients with renal cancer have an 11% to 13% risk of the cancer spreading to the brain. Leptomeningeal cancer may have normal imaging and will be diagnosed by malignant cells in the cerebrospinal fluid.

GROUP THERAPY AND CANCER

As alluded to earlier, group therapy has been shown to reduce stress and improve mortality in patients with cancer. In a very important study, Living Beyond Limits, done by David Spiegel and his associates at Stanford, women with metastatic breast cancer were randomized to receive weekly supportive group therapy for 1 year with medical treatment versus medical treatment only. The group therapy cohort had less mood disturbances, fewer phobic responses, and survived an average of 36.6 months compared to 19 months for the control group. In another study by Fawzy, newly diagnosed patients with malignant melanoma were randomized to participate in either a 6-week psychoeducational experience or a control group. The psychoeducational group had less psychological turmoil and significantly fewer subsequent deaths.

THE PSYCHIATRIST'S ROLE IN SMOKING CESSATION

Thirty percent of all cancer deaths and 87% of all lung cancer deaths are related to smoking. It has been shown that there is an increased rate of smoking among women and minorities, a fact that may be linked to the increased rate of cancer in these groups. While many long-time smokers believe that quitting won't reverse the damage they've already done, research has shown that, depending on the type of cancer, the mortality rate can drop 30–50% in former smokers as soon as 5 years after cessation. Unfortunately, only approximately one third of smokers make a serious annual attempt to quit and only 2.5% of all smokers succeed in achieving abstinence for 1 year.

Approximately 85% of people who successfully stop smoking appear to use one of the following methods: the "cold turkey" approach (abrupt cessation), gradual reduction, or a self-help group approach. The remainder use various techniques including replacement therapy with the nicotine patch or gum as well as adjunctive psychopharmacology treatment with bupropion (Wellbutrin or Zyban). Self-help groups and behavioral treatment, which include various modules, phone counseling, or scheduled smoking, all have been helpful. The C-L psychiatrist who works with cancer patients should be familiar with these various techniques so as to be able to discuss them in detail with patients. It is suggested that the patient's smoking status should be part of the "vital signs." One strategy to use is the four As model of smoking cessation (Ask about tobacco use, Advise to quit, Assist with a cessation plan, and Arrange follow-up and monitor progress). In scheduled smoking, a target date is selected and the patient smokes with varying frequencies, with or without reductions in the intercigarette interval. It is not unusual for a psychiatrist to teach patients various behavioral techniques as adjuncts for cessation of smoking. The ideal time to offer assistance in cessation of smoking is obviously before someone has developed cancer.

TUMOR MARKERS, GENETIC TESTING, AND SCREENING TECHNIQUES

A variety of new technologies have made it possible to identify individuals who are at a high risk for developing cancer. High-risk patients usually are counseled to alter behaviors, such as eating carcinogenic foods and excessive sun exposure, in order to delay the onset of disease.

Before genetic testing is undertaken, it is important to have a plan in place for pretest and posttest counseling. This will help identify patients with psychiatric disorders and those patients who are psychologically vulnerable to genetic testing. The model for this type of program is the approach to Huntington's disease, as well as the pre/post approach to testing that is utilized in human immunodeficiency virus (HIV) testing programs throughout the country. There are a few hereditary neoplastic gene traits and these include retinoblastoma, multiple endocrine neoplasia syndromes, and the hereditary breast and ovarian cancer familial syndrome due to mutations of the *BRCA1*. More is known about breast cancer gene testing than gene testing in other cancers. However, only 5% to 10% of cases of breast cancer seems to be strongly inherited. Testing positive for the mutation does not mean that the patient will definitely have breast or ovarian cancer.

Breast cancer screening with mammograms, prostate cancer screening with prostate-specific antigen (PSA), cervical cancer screening with pap smears, and colon cancer detection by colonoscopy are three widely used screening techniques. Patients who undergo such screening are rarely evaluated by a psychiatrist, unless a serious cancer is diagnosed. In working with such patients, we have found that false-positive test results can precipitate severe worry, which may take on an obsessive compulsive form, sometimes requiring psychiatric treatment. Mental health professionals also can help newly diagnosed patients deal with loss, despair, depression, anxiety, anger, and other strong emotions. The clinical task very well may be to help the patient understand that by having these tests, both patient and physician are providing the best possible chance for good health and are helping to minimize the negative consequences of unanticipated illness.

LIAISON POTENTIAL

1. Any specialized oncology unit has the potential for liaison work with a C-L psychiatrist. This approach typically includes the following activities:
   - Making work rounds with the oncology team at least once per week.
   - Attending and participating in weekly case conferences.
   - Regular meetings with social workers and nurse specialists assigned to the unit.
   - When feasible, doing preliminary consultation with inpatients or outpatients during the early phase of treatment so a relationship is established, if later interventions are needed.
2. Successful C-L liaison has been reported with many specialized cancer units. Examples are the following types of activities:
   - Bone marrow transplant programs where attention needs to be paid to the donors as well as the recipients.
   - Breast cancer treatment programs where there can be assistance in considering treatment options, genetic implications, and group therapy programs.
   - Ear, nose, and throat (ENT) cancer programs where psychological implications of disfiguring surgery are worked with as well as patients who have lost their vocal cords and will learn artificial speech.

3. Hospice programs and palliative care teams where patients with advanced cancer interface with specialized teams that should include a C-L psychiatrist.
4. The oncology staff, doctors, and nurses can experience distress when working with patients with cancer. They can have burnout. They often are receptive to meeting regularly to discuss individual cases or their own feelings. Sometimes, particularly nurses may wish to participate in a formal group meeting to discuss feelings and issues and/or learn various stress reduction techniques. Such formal groups seem to work best when they are time limited for several weeks to a year.

Psychonephrology

Essential Concepts

- Patients in renal failure (RF) often present with signs and symptoms of delirium.
- Depression and other affective disorders are the most common diagnoses in patients with renal disorders followed by delirium and dementia.
- Choice of dialysis type should take into account the patient's psychosocial situation.
- Most patients with RF who require psychotropic medication should not be given more than two-thirds of the maximum dose recommended for those with normal kidney function.
- Sexual dysfunction is common in patients on dialysis, in men in particular.

You know that you have passed muster as a consultation-liaison (C-L) psychiatrist when you have managed a few patients with RF. This group of patients is one of the most complex populations with whom C-L psychiatrists work. Apart from the various metabolic and physical variables that can complicate the picture, there is a whole gamut of confounding psychological issues related to RF, including renal transplantation, dialysis, and others. There is also a deceptive overlap of symptoms between depression and early RF. To top it off, RF itself can cause depressive syndromes.

CASE VIGNETTE: THE MAN WHO HAD MORE THAN THE FLU

A 38-year-old man presented to the psychiatric emergency room with delusional thinking that the Central Intelligence Agency (CIA) was following him.

He had been in good health, with no significant medical or psychiatric history until 3 months before admission, at which time he developed a flu-like syndrome with persistent fatigue. There were no medical findings, but, because of some marital problems, the patient was referred to psychotherapy with a psychologist who suggested that he speak with his general practitioner about antidepressant medication. The patient was prescribed fluoxetine (Prozac) (20 mg per day). He experienced some mild improvement in combined treatment, but his fatigue persisted, which was attributed to his depression. Three months later, over a period of a few days, he developed the above paranoid symptoms and was seen in a psychiatric emergency room. At that time, he also had a temperature of 101°F and, on physical examination; he had evidence of pneumonia that was confirmed by x-ray. The patient was admitted to the medical service and C-L consultation was called to follow-up the patient there. The following morning, when seen by the C-L consultant, he had a temperature of 103°F. The patient had full-blown delusional thinking that he was in a castle and was being chased by knights in armor. He had visual hallucinations, which were related to his delusion. He had difficulty concentrating and could not recall two out of three objects. His lab data showed white blood count (WBC) of 15,000, elevated blood urea nitrogen (BUN) of 50, and creatinine of 2.7. Urinalysis showed proteinuria.

The psychiatrist made a diagnosis of delirium secondary to renal disease. The patient was treated with haloperidol (Haldol), 1 mg twice a day. He was put on constant observation and given the supportive care protocol where staff would orient him regularly and the nightlight was kept on. He had a renal biopsy, which diagnosed Wegener's granuloma, an autoimmune disorder that affects the lungs and kidneys. The patient was put on peritoneal dialysis and switched to hemodialysis within a week. His mental status cleared within 48 hours of his first dialysis. Both the patient and his wife were receptive to discussion with the psychiatrist about the nature of his psychotic symptoms, which had been frightening to them and their children. They were periodically seen over the next several years, during which time the patient was switched to home dialysis and eventually had a renal transplant.

ACUTE RENAL FAILURE

RF should be included in the differential diagnosis in patients who present with fatigue and depression. The correct diagnosis is easier to make with patients who have a medical evaluation with appropriate tests, which should include blood creatinine and BUN, as well as urinalysis. With RF and the accumulation of toxic metabolites in the blood, the characteristic picture of delirium emerges. Mental status changes occur often in RF. These can range from subtle abnormalities in concentration and intelligence to marked confusion, lethargy, and myoclonus. Although some cognitive impairments are reversible with dialysis, others may persist. The etiology of acute mental status changes include a whole host of metabolic abnormalities, such as uremia, anemia, hypophosphatemia, hypoglycemia, hyperparathyroidism, as well as other nonmetabolic conditions, such as cerebrovascular disease, subdural hematomas, meningitis/encephalitis, drug intoxication, seizure disorder, and so on. As is often the case with delirium, it is essential to identify and treat the underlying cause of the delirium as well as treating the patient symptomatically. Low-dose haloperidol can be used to help control the agitation and reduce psychotic manifestations, until the RF is corrected by dialysis. Because haloperidol is detoxified in the liver, there is little risk in the use of this drug in appropriate doses in patients with RF. The atypical neuroleptics may also be helpful.

Diagnosing Delirium Due to a Medical Condition

The patient must have each of the following [from Diagnostic and Statistical Manual of Mental Disorders-IV (DSM-IV)]:

1. Disturbance of consciousness with reduced clarity of awareness of the environment and reduced ability to focus, sustain, or shift attention.
2. A change in cognition (such as memory deficit, disorientation, or language disturbance) or the development of a perceptual disturbance that is not better accounted for by a preexisting, established, or evolving dementia.
3. The disturbance develops over a short period of time (usually hours to days) and tends to fluctuate during the course of the day.

4. There is evidence from the history, physical examination, or laboratory findings that the disturbance is caused by the direct physiological consequences of a general medical condition.

CHRONIC RENAL FAILURE AND DIALYSIS

In the past, RF virtuously always had a fatal prognosis, which is probably why it had been called *end-stage renal disease* (*ESRD*). Modern scientific advances have made available various forms of dialysis, in which kidney function is artificially maintained. There is also the possibility of renal transplantation, which has progressed to the point where nonrelated donors can provide the organ. Although these techniques will prolong and save lives, all patients with RF can still have many psychological issues. The patient's responses to the need for chronic dialysis are many and varied. The very fact that one has to depend on dialysis to maintain life is a major stressor by itself. Consider, too, the independence lost by the patient and the dependence on machines that could possibly malfunction at any time. Coping mechanisms of chronic dialysis patients include denial, regression, aggression, and depression. There are, of course, those people who have a mature acceptance of their condition. The interaction between the staff and the patient also influences the emotional state of the patient. Therefore, liaison work between the staff and the renal patient is a continuous dynamic process.

The choice of the form of dialysis ideally should take into account medical factors, the availability of resources, and the patients' psychosocial state, in particular their independency needs. Those patients who have a great need for independence should be considered for self-care center dialysis, home hemodialysis or peritoneal dialysis, or a renal transplant. Input from you may be helpful to the nephrology team in making their recommendation as to the best type of dialysis for a particular patient. Some psychotherapeutic work with the patient also may help the patient realize what type of dialysis he or she would prefer.

Hemodialysis is typically performed three times a week for approximately 4 to 6 hours each session either at a dialysis center in the community or in a hospital or at home. The patient sits in a comfortable chair and is connected to the dialysis machine through tubing into a surgically created fistula that is usually in the patient's forearm. If all goes well, the patient can read or watch television during the "dialysis run." In past years, there were frequent episodes of hypotension and other complications, as alarms from the machines would sound. Now these are rare and most dialysis sessions are uneventful. Nevertheless, many patients find it difficult to make adjustments in their lifestyles in order to accommodate the requirements of hemodialysis.

Home dialysis, as the name implies, occurs in the home and requires a family member to learn how to administer it and be with the patient. This can put great stress on the family member who is responsible for running the dialysis. Although remote, there is the possibility of a medical emergency that they have to be trained to handle, and there is generally a major impact on the family member's day-to-day schedule. The family dynamics can become an important factor in the success of this type of treatment.

Continuous ambulatory peritoneal dialysis (CAPD) is another option. Typically, patients have a surgically implanted catheter that allows access to the peritoneal cavity and then self-administers dialysis through gravity flow several times during the day for brief periods or continuously throughout the night. While this method allows for more freedom and freer food restriction, because the patient is not tied to a dialysis machine, the likelihood of infections is higher. The patient must use meticulous techniques if infections are to be avoided with CAPD. Also, patients on CAPD can gain weight and have a bloated abdomen, which may not be acceptable to them.

CASE VIGNETTE: THE COUPLE WHO FINISHED EACH OTHER'S SENTENCES

A 38-year-old married man required being on dialysis because of RF. C-L consultation was requested while the patient was in the hospital during the acute phase of his illness because his wife insisted on being present with her husband past visiting hours. They had been married 10 years and both described a very close and happy marriage. When interviewed together, they would finish each other's sentences. At one point, when the patient could not remember a dream that he had before he came into the hospital, his wife reported it in great detail. She would refer to her husband's illness as "our kidney disease."

They noted that every purchase, no matter how large or small, was always made jointly. On the basis of information from the C-L consultant, a mutual decision was made for the patient to be on home dialysis.

The patient and his wife were seen in periodic follow-up over the next few years. The home dialysis appeared to work quite well as the wife was able to skillfully manage the three times per week procedure. The husband continued working for a major corporation and would have dialysis in the late afternoon and would often help his children with their homework during the dialysis. Because dialysis worked so well and there were no family members who matched for transplant, such an option was put on hold.

In the fifth year, during a follow up-visit, it was noted that there was subtle marital discord and there appeared to be hostility previously absent between the couple. During an individual meeting with the wife, she noted that she was going to graduate school and wanted to work at least part time. She felt stifled by the obligation of always being available to do the dialysis. She believed that her own life was not going anywhere, whereas her husband, despite his illness, was progressing in his career. A series of discussions were held with the couple and with each of them individually. They were able to discuss the arrangement between the two of them and they made a decision to go on center dialysis. Ultimately, the patient put his name on the list for a cadaver transplant.

Quality of Life Issues and Dialysis

Because of the restrictions posed by dialysis, there are marked differences in the quality of life, depending on the treatment used. Patients who have had successful transplants do better than those on peritoneal or hemodialysis. Depression is common in this population (6% to 34% prevalence rate) and can be affected by other medical conditions or by medications. If allowed to persist, depressive symptoms are associated with a higher mortality and more frequent hospitalizations.

Sexual dysfunction is a frequent complication in patients on dialysis. In men, this may take the form of erectile dysfunction, whereas women often experience altered menstrual cycles and decreased libido. For some, function may return at least partially after a successful transplant. The loss of the ability to urinate in male patients also may contribute to this problem, as do depression medications and endocrine changes. Although this issue is quite significant to the patient, often it is ignored by medical staff. Treatment of sexual dysfunction includes medication sexual counseling and in some cases implantation of a penile prosthesis. The use of sildenafil (Viagra) and other phosphodiesterase inhibitors have been shown to be between 60% and 80% efficacious for erectile dysfunction and is widely used by men on dialysis. Although you may be tempted to offer a patient with erectile dysfunction a trial of sildenafil, be careful to rule out underlying cardiac disease because of the danger of the synergistic effect with nitrates that are used to treat angina that may lower blood pressure to dangerous levels.

Withdrawal/discontinuation of dialysis accounts for approximately 20% to 25% of deaths of patients on dialysis. This happens because patients on dialysis often develop increasing medical complications that may severely affect their quality of life. A psychiatric consultation should be obtained in patients who request the termination of dialysis. Ultimately, a large number of patients do decide that they do not want to continue. Obviously, an assessment of the patient's mental state should be made to determine that the patient is not confused and does understand the implications of this life-ending decision. Major depression should be ruled out. Oftentimes, the patient is not depressed, but is just considering his or her quality of life realistically. Patients who rationally decide to withdraw treatment are usually older than 60 years of age and have other chronic diseases, such as diabetes. After discontinuation of dialysis, the average patient lives for 8 to 12 days.

As a C-L psychiatrist, you may find yourself in the middle of a very delicate situation in which a rational competent patient wants to stop dialysis, while the family and/or the dialysis team disagrees. The patient may not have the capacity to make such a decision because of delirium or dementia. The family may have the patient's living will or may declare that they are aware of the patient's wishes in this situation. Your main role usually is to determine if a mental illness, such as delirium, dementia, or depression, is interfering with the patient's capacity to make such a decision. In most states, a court then takes over. Hospital ethics committees can be useful in these situations and may meet with the treating team, the family, and the psychiatrist. The renal community recognizes and recommends the role of palliative care in the end-of-life treatment of patients.

CASE VIGNETTE: THE WOMAN WHO DID NOT MEAN "NO"

An 82-year-old Italian-speaking grandmother with a very dedicated and loving large family was on center hemodialysis because of RF. She was viewed as having been depressed for approximately 2 years and frequently would be reluctant to come for her three times per week dialysis run. She had been on Prozac for approximately 1 year with no apparent change. Most recently, the patient's fistula clotted and there were no more readily available sites. Surgery was recommended to create a vascular site for dialysis and the patient refused to go along with this procedure. The family explained that she had suffered enough and now just wanted to stop the dialysis and peacefully pass away. The first C-L consultant interviewed the patient with the family as translator and also understood enough Italian to confirm that this was what the patient was requesting. There was no evidence of significant depression or overt psychosis. The family was very sad about this decision, but felt strongly about respecting her wishes.

A second C-L consultant came to see the patient, but, rather than use the family as translators or have them be present during the interview, he asked a nursing supervisor who spoke Italian to do this task. The patient related well and showed a clear sensorium, very much aware of her surroundings and situation. The patient noted that she did not want to die and enjoyed being at home visiting with her grandchildren and watching television. She was not in significant discomfort. However, she believed that her children believed it was time for her to move on. She wrongly believed that her medical care was a financial burden to her family. She also believed that family members who brought her for dialysis were taking valuable time away from their jobs and family and even could give some examples of things they had said to confirm this. She believed that the surgery to establish her dialysis site was very unusual and that the doctors resented doing it. Therefore, she thought that the right thing to do was to refuse the procedure and peacefully die. She viewed the family as respecting her statement that she did not want dialysis as proof that she was a burden.

The C-L psychiatrist needed to do some sensitive delicate follow-up work with the patient and family to get the patient to accept the surgical procedure and continue on dialysis. The family arranged a rotating schedule of drivers for her dialysis that included the grandchildren, which proved to be very gratifying for all those concerned.

Neuropsychiatric syndromes on dialysis—There are two specific dialysis-related neuropsychiatric syndromes that you should recognize: dysequilibrium syndrome and dialysis dementia.

Dysequilibrium syndrome is a transient delirious state that usually includes headaches, nausea, irritability, muscle cramps, agitation, drowsiness, seizures, and occasionally psychotic symptoms that occur in the third or fourth hour of dialysis or approximately 8 to 48 hours after completion of dialysis. This syndrome usually occurs in patients who have been undergoing rapid dialysis and is caused by overcorrection of metabolic abnormalities. The nephrologist usually is aware of this situation and treats the abnormality although there may be a lag period between treatment of the metabolic abnormality and the disappearance of the symptoms.

Dialysis dementia is a rare syndrome that is characterized by progressive encephalopathy, stuttering, dysarthria, dysphasia, myoclonic jerks, paranoia, depression, and seizures. This syndrome occurs in patients who have been undergoing chronic hemodialysis, and the etiology appears to be related to aluminum toxicity and can be fatal. Although prevalent in the past, the incidence has decreased, due to the use of aluminum-free dialysate. There is no known treatment.

Treatment Approach to Delirium and Dementia Syndromes in ESRD

1. Determine underlying etiology and attempt to reverse or alleviate disease process.
2. Treat agitation or acute psychosis with low dosage of neuroleptic, such as Haldol (0.25 to 1 mg b.i.d.

by mouth titrating upward as indicated), with intra-muscular (IM) or intravenous (IV) routes to be considered in special circumstances.

3. Atypical antipsychotics may have a role here; to be determined by clinical experience and new literature and research.

4. Adjunct use of lorazepam (Ativan) can be used to control symptoms.

5. Most patients with RF who require psychotropic medication should not receive more than two-thirds of the maximum dose recommended for those with normal kidney function (Table 4.1).

6. Constant observation and limited use of restraints should be considered for any psychotic or confused patient who could be dangerous to himself or herself or others.

7. Frequent reorientation techniques and night light should be utilized.

8. Explain nature of the condition to family and to the patient after recovery.

RENAL TRANSPLANT

Generally speaking, renal transplantation is a desirable for most patients as it enables them to live a relatively normal life because it improves renal functioning. There are two types of organ donations: living donors (who can be related or non-related) and cadaveric donors. Psychiatrists and other mental health clinicians often are involved in the process of donor selection because there are so many psychosocial issues that arise in the process. As you do your evaluations, questions to ask include the following: Is family coercion involved? Is a potential donor harboring resentment, while appearing superficially altruistic? Factors that affect the outcome of renal transplantation include graft rejection, side effects of immunosuppressant drugs (particularly, neuropsychiatric side effects), and the possibility of disease recurrence, as well as psychosocial concerns. Psychiatric modalities include brief supportive therapy, pharmacologic interventions, and behavioral interventions. The ideal situation is to have a liaison psychiatrist as part of the team, from the donor selection process up to the postoperative stage.

TABLE 4.1. Neuropsychiatric Effects of Psychotrophic
Medication Used in End Stage Renal
Disease/Transplantation

Medication	Comments
	"*The rule of two-thirds*" is recommended, even if the drug does not affect renal function
Lithium	Contraindicated in *acute* renal failure, but can be used in chronic renal failure
	Completely dialyzed, recommendation is to decrease to 300–600 mg and give as a single dose postdialysis
	Decrease dose in patients on cyclosporine
Neuroleptics	Haldol and phenothiazines not dialyzable
	No dose modification required
	Phenothiazines not recommended (sedation, urinary retention, and orthostatic hypotension)
Tricyclic anti depressants	Those with hydroxylated metabolites are markedly elevated in renal disease
	Nortriptyline useful secondary to therapeutic window
	Amitriptyline, imipramine, and desipramine are <6% excreted through the kidneys
	Nortriptyline and doxepin half-lives are increased in RF
Selective serotonin reuptake inhibitor	Fluoxetine is highly protein bound. It also has a long half-life; may need to adjust dose
	Paroxetine concentration is increased in decreased renal function
	Follow rule of two-thirds for all of the SSRIs
Other anti depressants	Electrolyte imbalances in RF may potentiate seizures in patients on bupropion
	Clearance of venlafaxine is decreased in renal disease; need dose adjustment
	Monoamine oxidase inhibitors (MAOIs) cause orthostatic hypotension, especially after dialysis

TABLE 4.1. *Continued*

Medication	Comments
Anxiolytics/sedative hypnotics	Barbiturates can increase osteomalacia; also increased sedation
	Alprazolam, chlordiazepoxide, and diazepam have active metabolites; cause increased psychomotor effects
	Chloral hydrate not contraindicated, but avoid when glomerular filtration rate <50 mL/min
	Lorazepam, oxazepam, temazepam, and klonopin are not dialyzable, but half-life is increased in RF
	Buspirone half-life is increased in RF; needs dose reduction
Anti convulsants	Valproate can be used
	Carbamazepine has antidiuretic action, not dialyzable; preferred over phenobarbital and phenytoin in patients with seizures

RF, renal failure.

PSYCHOPHARMACOLOGY IN RENAL DISEASE

Most psychotropic medications, except lithium, are metabolized in the liver and not the kidney. Therefore, technically, there is no need for dose adjustment. However, in real life, renal patients are quite vulnerable to the adverse side effects. This may be related to lower levels of protein for drug binding. Therefore, a clinical rule of thumb is that one should not give more than two-thirds of the maximum dose recommended for people with normal kidney function. When prescribing psychotropics to renal patients, pay close attention to drug–drug interactions.

Neuroleptics—There is no need for dose modification. We must remember that haloperidol and phenothiazines are not dialyzable, but this does not mean that they cannot be given to patients on dialysis. Phenothiazines, such as thorazine, are not well tolerated because of anticholinergic side effects, particularly orthostatic hypotension and sedation. In general, starting doses are lower than usual and high potency neuroleptics appear to be well tolerated. Atypical antipsychotics are well tolerated in this population.

Antidepressants—The role of tricyclic antidepressants (TCAs) have been studied more extensively in patients with RF, compared to other antidepressants. However, all antidepressants can probably be used. Nortriptyline, with its well-defined therapeutic window, is preferred among the TCAs. Selective serotonin reuptake inhibitors (SSRIs) and other antidepressants are prescribed quite commonly, although they have not been as thoroughly studied in renal disease. One of us (MB) participated in research that established the efficacy and safety of fluoxetine in patients with ESRD. When using fluoxetine, it is useful to remember that it is highly protein bound and, as such, can displace warfarin (Coumadin) and digoxin, among other medications that renal patients are often prescribed. In general, we have found SSRIs to be quite safe in renal patients, although we recommend careful monitoring for side effects. We recommend caution when using bupropion in patients with RF because electrolyte imbalances often make them more vulnerable to seizures. Monoamine oxidase inhibitors (MAOIs) also can be useful, particularly in patients who are refractory. However, we need to keep in mind that these cause orthostatic hypotension, which is also a common postdialysis phenomenon (Table 4.1).

Antianxiety agents—We recommend that you use benzodiazepines, with no active metabolites, to prevent the possibility of accumulation in patients with RF. These include clonazepam, lorazepam, oxazepam, or temazepam. Buspirone, a nonbenzodiazepine anxiolytic that is given on a continuous basis, is metabolized in the liver and may also be used. SSRIs also should be considered as antianxiety agents.

Lithium—Be cautious when using lithium in patients with renal disease. Assess kidney function both before and during lithium therapy. Although lithium is contraindicated in acute RF, it may be used in chronic RF. Although lithium therapy can impair renal concentrating ability in healthy people, it may be used in RF, among other reasons, because of the lack of functioning kidneys. Lithium may be used in people with RF because it is ordinarily solely removed by the kidneys, but entirely removed by dialysis treatment. It should be given in the dialysate during peritoneal dialysis or given as a single oral dose after each hemodialysis treatment.

TABLE 4.2. Neuropsychiatric Complications
of Medications Used in Renal Diseases

Corticosteroids	Euphoria, mania, psychosis, depression
Anabolic steroids	Paranoia, mania, depression, aggressive behavior
Reserpine	Depression
Methyldopa	Confusion, depression, dementia
Prazosin	Drowsiness, depression, nervousness
Thiazides	Weakness, pseudodepression
Clonidine	Depression, hallucinations
Ace inhibitors	Depression, somnolence, insomnia, nervousness
Calcium channel blockers	Depression
Ondansetron	Panic, fear, agitation, emotional lability
Cyclosporine	Confusion
Beta blockers	Depression

Anticonvulsants—In patients with preexisting seizure disorder, carbamazepine, valproic acid, and the newer
anticonvulsant drugs, such as topiramate, lamotrigine,
and gabapentin, can be used. They are also alternatives to
lithium in patients who have bipolar affective disorders or
impulse control disorders. Carbamazepine is not dialyzable
and is preferred over phenobarbital and phenytoin, for this
reason. However, the newer anticonvulsants are probably
safe to use and have better side effect profiles, although
they are not as well studied.

LIAISON POTENTIAL

1. Patients on dialysis often have chronic medical problems (Table 4.2) that interfere with quality of life and
   lead to many psychosocial issues. They have a therapeutic
   relationship with the renal team that is made up of nephrologists, dialysis nurses, and social workers, who often are
   quite receptive to having C-L psychiatrists attend case
   conferences and rounds, meet with staff, and see patients
   often during their regularly scheduled dialysis runs.
2. Renal transplant programs are ideal for liaison work by C-L
   psychiatrists. There is value in having a full psychosocial
   evaluation before the transplant to anticipate the type of

adjustment problems that patients will have. Resistance to full compliance with medication and diet often has a complicated psychological basis. These issues are best discussed as part of a team effort that includes team meetings and liaison work.
3. Meetings with family members individually and in groups can be helpful, and is often done in coordination with other members of the psychosocial team, such as social workers and dialysis nurses. Seeing donating family members before and after transplant can be a valuable contribution.
4. Regular rounds with the nephrologists, entire renal team, transplant team, and intensive care unit (ICU) team are traditional liaison activities that have had a favorable impact on patients on dialysis.

ACKNOWLEDGEMENT

The authors would like to thank Norman B. Levy, MD, for his help in revising this chapter.

Psychological Care of the Burn and Trauma Patient

Essential Concepts

- Patients with trauma and burn injuries are frequently undermedicated for pain.
- Patients treated with narcotics for pain after a trauma or burn injury rarely become physically dependent on the pain medication, but staff, patients, and families frequently are fearful that they will become so.
- Flashbacks, intrusive thoughts, and dreams of the accident are frequent sequelae after accidents and will usually diminish in frequency over the following days and weeks.
- Amputations, loss of function, and scarring of the face and genitals have a serious psychological impact on patients and should not be minimized, despite any initial denial by the patient of psychological symptoms.

Trauma and burn injuries occur suddenly, without warning. In a few seconds, a person's life often is changed forever. The psychological and psychiatric impact of such injuries is apparent almost immediately and has far-reaching and long-term implications. The accompanying physical pain takes center stage and must be dealt with before the finer psychological points can be addressed. Symptoms of acute stress and then posttraumatic stress frequently become part of the clinical picture and need to be recognized and treated. The individual psychological response to each of these issues is complicated by problems, such as substance abuse, amputations, loss of function, and scarring, when they occur.

PAIN AND PAIN CONTROL

As a novice consultation-liaison (C-L) consultant seeing a trauma or burn patient, you may have unrealistic expectations. You may assume that your patient will want to discuss the trauma and the variety of emotions and psychological conflicts that it triggered. But, at first, the only issue that your patient cares about is pain and pain control. Until this issue is recognized and addressed, all other concerns will be discussed in the most superficial and transient manner.

Each time you see your patient during the acute phase of injury, ask about his or her pain control and how he or she is handling it. Your notes should comment on the degree of apparent pain control and the patient's satisfaction. As a psychiatric consultant, you should be particularly knowledgeable about pain control, including specific medications with equianalgesic dosages, onset of action, side effects, and drug interactions. Especially when the medical/surgery treatment team is not knowledgeable about pain control or there is no pain consultant, the psychiatrist will need to step up and fill this role.

PSYCHOLOGICAL REACTIONS TO TRAUMA AND BURN

A trauma or a burn injury is almost always an unexpected event. Even people who have dangerous jobs, such as police or fire personnel, do not expect to be seriously injured and are not psychologically prepared for trauma. Similarly, the person who has made a suicide attempt does not anticipate the aftermath of the injury.

The initial psychological response will be colored by the intensity of pain and the effectiveness of pain management. During the acute phase of a severe injury, there is often an initial period of psychological withdrawal. This is more likely to occur with a large burn, loss of limb, or serious threat to life, although the reaction is common to most injured people, particularly children. The withdrawn patient shows little interest in external events, family, or friends. The patient's affect is often blunted, which may seem paradoxical in the setting of a major injury in which great concern might be expected. This is often mistaken for depression, but, in fact, the patient rarely communicates true depressive ideation, loss of self-esteem, grieving, or guilty feelings at this point. This response is probably due to a combination of two factors: a physiological phenomenon called *conservation-withdrawal* and the defense mechanism of denial.

Conservation-withdrawal is due to an activation of the parasympathetic system with decreased heart rate, blood pressure, body temperature, muscle tone, and general motor activity. It usually subsides within 1 to 2 weeks, but can last longer if there is a sustained physiological threat to the patient's life.

Denial is a protective unconscious defense mechanism that relieves anxiety that arises when an individual is threatened by the possibility of death, mutilation, and pain. Denial not only reduces anxiety but it also reduces the catecholamine response, triggered by anxiety, which may protect the cardio-vascular system. Our medical and surgical colleagues may see denial as a pathological process that is based on unreality and they may ask us to remove it. However, the abrupt removal of denial in the early phase of an injury may disrupt a vulnerable ego, leading to marked anxiety, a narcissistic rage, severe depression, and even overt psychosis. Patients in denial often will resist receiving information about their condition. We recommend providing such information in small doses and infrequently. Usually in the 1 or 2 weeks after pain is in control, the denial will give way to reasonable reality testing. It may, however, take many months or sometimes longer before a severely injured person fully understands and accepts new limitations.

Anxiety is a universal response to all illness, especially when strong denial is not operating, but it takes on particular characteristics at the time of trauma and burn. Under these circumstances, the patient no longer perceives himself or herself as being fully intact. The sense of wholeness is violated. This can create almost overwhelming anxiety and, at times, a psychotic decompensation.

Another cause of anxiety in trauma patients is separation anxiety. From a psychodynamic point of view, this type of anxiety is believed to have its origin during early childhood, when the child is struggling with separation from the mother. The practical value of such a formulation is that it may alert you to appreciating why some people who had problems with separation as a child may have difficulty at the time of a sudden forced hospitalization.

Although you will understandably bring a psychological mindset to most of your consultations, think differently if called to the bedside to see a posttrauma patient who has had some broken bones and now has overwhelming anxiety, shortness of breath, and fear that he or she is dying. Although it may be a panic attack, do not miss an acute pulmonary embolism, which presents exactly like this.

Depression is to be expected in response to an injury that involves loss of body function and loss of family and work roles. Your patient may verbalize sadness, may weep, or may simply have a sad facial expression. Diminished appetite, weight loss, sleep disturbances, early morning awakenings, and decreased psychomotor activity are hallmarks of a major depression. However, it may be difficult to diagnose a depressed state by vegetative signs alone because the injury (particularly burn injuries) may bring about some of these symptoms in the absence of depression.

Similarly, it may be difficult to distinguish grief from major depression. Generally speaking, the nondepressed grieving patient does not have a significant decrease in self-esteem. The patient realizes that the injury has caused some losses and limitations, but does not feel less lovable as a person and has not lost the belief that he or she deserves the affection and attention of others. We begin to consider that the injured person has progressed to a serious depression when there is a concomitant decrease in the patient's sense of worthiness as a person. Instead of a preoccupation with memories, sadness about loss, and rumination about real issues, the more seriously depressed patient begins to give the loss a meaning that damages self-esteem. For example, the amputee views himself or herself as "just a cripple" or the burned patient views himself or herself as a "disfigured nobody."

ACUTE STRESS AND POSTTRAUMATIC STRESS SYMPTOMS

Most traumatic injuries occur in situations that fulfill Diagnostic and Statistical Manual of Mental Disorders, Fourth Edition (DSM-IV) criteria for a "traumatic event": an event that involves "actual or threatened death or serious injury or a threat to the physical integrity of self or others." The patient's response usually involves intense fear and sometimes helplessness or horror. These are the two most important criteria for both acute stress disorder and post-traumatic stress disorder (PTSD). In our experience, severely injured patients will meet criteria for the diagnosis of acute stress disorder. When these symptoms last for at least 1 month, the diagnosis of PTSD is made.

From a practical point of view, as a consultant, you should be less concerned with making an official diagnosis than with recognizing which symptoms can be treated. Pay particular attention to flashbacks, nightmares, and situations that remind the patient of the accident and bring on anxiety. Usually there is gradual improvement of these symptoms with time and you can monitor this improvement. Failure to show a stepwise improvement, usually over a 1- to 2-week period, usually indicates the need for more intensive psychotherapy, often with the addition of medications.

PSYCHOTHERAPY AND PSYCHOPHARMACOLOGY IN THE TRAUMA SETTING

Specific techniques of psychotherapy are discussed in detail in Chapter 16. For most patients, some review of the circumstances of the accident will be helpful. Where there are persistent symptoms, you may need to undertake a more detailed debriefing of the incident. In this situation, you should not only review memories of the traumatic event and any accompanying emotions, but you also should explore the patient's associations to the incident and the interplay with other conflicts that the patient may have. The pace of making any therapeutic intervention should be based on your assessment of the patient's ego strength, and ability to cope with such material without being overwhelmed.

Anxiety symptoms may be treated with psychopharmacology, as well as with relaxation techniques or hypnosis, in some situations. It bears repeating that pain control is of prime importance and, without it, no anxiety treatment is likely to be effective.

With regard to benzodiazepines, we tend to favor clonazepam (Klonopin). It has a half-life of approximately 15 hours and it can be used once or twice a day. Rarely do you see "clock-watching," nor are there sudden episodes of anxiety in between dosages. The dosage can be started at 0.5 mg and can be cut in half or titrated up, as needed. It is also relatively easy to taper the dosage when the decision is made to discontinue the medication.

Sertraline (Zoloft) has been approved by the U.S. Food and Drug Administration (FDA) for the treatment of PTSD. We believe that the other selective serotonin reuptake inhibitors

(SSRIs) are equally effective for PTSD. We suggest, however, that you use medications as part of a multifaceted approach that includes psychotherapeutic intervention.

Recall that a trauma or burn injury does not occur in a vacuum. Each of your patients will have a specific psychological makeup that will influence the psychological response to the trauma. As part of this, your patient will likely have specific fantasies about why and how he or she was injured. During your assessment, ask about meaningful things that may have led up to the injury or that may have happened after the incident.

CASE VIGNETTE: EXPECTED TRAUMA?

A 55-year-old man severely injured his right arm in a printing press accident. He was overheard by the hospital staff to say that he "expected something like this to happen sooner or later." An inquiry into the meaning of this statement by the C-L consultant revealed that he expected it not only because his employer did not maintain the printing press equipment adequately, but also because he felt he deserved to be punished for something that had happened more than 35 years ago. As a teenager, while driving while intoxicated, he had caused an auto accident in which one person was killed and another was paralyzed.

Traumatic amputations can occur at time of the accident or can occur in necessary surgery subsequent to the trauma. There are very important psychosocial implications of amputation as well as situations where there is reimplantation. These topics are covered in Chapter 11.

LIAISON POTENTIAL

1. Specialized trauma centers or emergency rooms offer an ideal setting for a C-L psychiatrist to connect.
2. The liaison effort here would usually involve working with other mental health professionals in seeing family members who receive sudden notification of death and injury.

3. Similarly, a burn unit should have a C-L psychiatrist working with the social worker and clinical nurse specialist who see patients and families.

4. Working together with the trauma, burn, or emergency room team is often essential as patients deal with shock of sudden injury and life-threatening injuries.

5. The C-L psychiatrist can provide valuable liaison to an ethics team or ethics committee concerning the patient's state of mind when momentous life or death decisions are being made.

6. Patients who have undergone amputation and/or replantation often are treated by a team of doctors and nurses who would benefit from having a C-L psychiatrist work with them.

7. Regular rounds with house staff and nurses of a burn and trauma unit usually will be greatly appreciated. There is often a *esprit de corps* among such staff and they will welcome another professional who is dedicated to working in this area.

6

Psychological Care of the Obstetric Patient

Essential Concepts

- There is a clear role for the consultation-liaison (C-L) psychiatrist in the case of a pregnant woman who has hyperemesis gravidarum, enforced bed rest, or substance abuse.
- The so-called unwanted pregnancy often reflects conscious and unconscious conflicts and ambivalence of either partner.
- Women with schizophrenia are at risk for decompensation prenatally and postpartum.
- There are appropriate situations where certain psychotropic medications can be used effectively and safely during pregnancy.
- Postpartum psychosis can occur 1 to 2 weeks after delivery and usually requires hospitalization because of potential suicidality and concern about infanticide.

Pregnancy and delivery are generally a joyous period in a woman's life. However, much can go wrong and any complication can be accompanied with much emotional suffering and loss of self-worth. Your role as a C-L psychiatrist is to help the patient through a major life crisis, which also can promote the well-being of an unborn or newborn child. In this chapter, we address psychological issues that arise throughout the cycle of conception, pregnancy, and childbirth.

CONCEPTION

Infertility occurs in approximately 5% to 10% of couples. Although coping with this problem can bring a couple closer together, it also can lead to increased conflict that may require marital counseling or individual therapy. The man may feel "less of a man" and be reluctant to have his sperm tested. Women who have difficulty conceiving may feel unfeminine or worthless. Sometimes there is extreme guilt about any previous abortions.

New reproductive technology can allow artificial insemination, surrogate pregnancy, or other variations using gamete and embryo transfers. Some of these techniques require hormonal injections to the woman that can cause mood changes, especially when they are abruptly stopped. There sometimes has to be "sex on demand" at a particular time, which causes tension and, at times, performance anxiety with potential impotency problems. When a woman becomes pregnant after a long and arduous process, there can be great elation. However, this can be followed by a letdown and even depression as the symptoms of pregnancy and/or the tasks of caring for a newborn bring the couple down a notch. When there are difficulties here, early psychiatric consultation and intervention may be helpful. In fact, many fertility specialists refer patients for psychotherapy as an integral part of their treatment. Patients may need not only treatment of anxiety and depression but also the opportunity to explore issues of guilt and blame, as well as distortions of body image.

UNWANTED PREGNANCY

It is a reasonable question in the interview of a pregnant woman to ask if the pregnancy was planned. If the pregnancy is acknowledged as unplanned, we suggest you inquire into the circumstances of the pregnancy and the details of any failed method of birth control. From our experience, it is quite rare that the patient did not have proper education or information about proper birth control. A careful case history may reveal the life circumstances that brought about a conscious or unconscious desire to have a baby and therefore to expose herself to the possibility of a pregnancy. For example, a woman might "run out of birth control pills" and/or "forget to renew the prescription." Or perhaps a woman will decide to "take a chance" and not insert her intrauterine device (IUD) or will believe her cycle is not in the fertile period, and therefore will agree to let her partner not use condoms.

Frequently, in all of these types of situations, you will find that the patient had mixed feelings about becoming pregnant. For example, a woman may have just visited a relative or a friend with young children and was thinking about wanting to have a baby when she failed to use her usual method of birth control. You also should consider carefully the role of the male partner in the so-called unwanted pregnancy. For example, coitus interruptus (withdrawal), a method of birth control that often fails, is a method in which the male can determine the successful or unsuccessful outcome. Either partner may have a need to prolong the relationship by bringing about a pregnancy, even if it was not previously discussed and planned. The conflict, which may have led to a pregnancy, has the potential to undermine any marital or partner relationship, influence future parent–child relationship, and bring about future repeated unwanted pregnancies. Even when an unwanted pregnancy is accepted, it may be helpful to suggest psychotherapy to deal with the underlying conflicts.

COMPLICATIONS DURING PREGNANCY

Hyperemesis gravidarum—*Hyperemesis gravidarum* is a potential complication of pregnancy that occurs in approximately 1 to 3 cases per 1,000 births. The exact cause of nausea and vomiting has not been established. It is believed to be related to the level of human chorionic gonadotropic hormone, which tends to be high in the blood and urine during the first 12 weeks of gestation. This corresponds to the usual duration of nausea and vomiting during management of diet (frequent smaller meals and certain bland foods, such as crackers and dry toast) and avoidance of triggers (odors and certain foods). When vomiting is complicated by dehydration, intravenous (IV) fluids and correction of electrolytes may be necessary. Certain antiemetics, including metoclopramide, have been used and, to date, have not been associated with reproductive complications.

Disruptions to the lifestyle of the mother who has this condition are many and far-reaching. The mother may have to go on leave from work much sooner than expected or have to abruptly quit school. She may be unable to leave the house and may face multiple hospitalizations. Some women have described a sense of isolation and vulnerability in which control has been taken away from them physically, emotionally, and even financially. Others have described a loss of desirability, feeling surrounded by "spit-up" cups, and constantly having foul breath. This is one condition in which feelings about the pregnancy may be very different from those about the baby. Hospitalized patients have, at times, expressed uncertainty as to whether they can go on with the pregnancy, fantasizing about preterm delivery, although the baby is very much wanted. In rare cases, patients have opted for termination, especially in the earliest weeks when the vomiting tends to be the most severe. A supportive nonjudgmental approach is crucial for all involved because this condition is very painful and can become life threatening. Interventions such as supportive therapy, visiting nurse services, and guided relaxation can be helpful. There also may be times when psychotropic medications are needed to address sleep disturbances, depression, or severe anxiety related to this condition.

Bed rest—There are multiple conditions in which the recommended treatment involves bed rest, including preterm labor, preeclampsia, premature rupture of the membranes, placenta previa, and severe hypertension. The strictness of the bed rest can vary from the patient being hospitalized for months with minimal movement and no bathroom privileges to a regime where the patient is at home and may walk around occasionally. Again, however, even with "lighter" restrictions, the disruption to the lifestyle and work can be severe.

Some women have described bed rest as a sort of voluntary incarceration, with the prison cell being the size of a bed. Aggravating the physical stress is the ongoing awareness that, at any point, there could be a precipitous delivery that leads to loss or compromise of the baby. Other women have described a combined sense of helplessness and guilt, blaming themselves or their bodies at times for not having a "normal" pregnancy. Still others have expressed a sense of being cheated after all of their efforts and devotion to becoming parents. These feelings often are compounded when there are young children at home.

When bed rest is prolonged, the emotional and physical demands on the mother can seem extreme. In these cases, supportive interventions from you and the staff will be very important in validating the mother's experience and helping her to "carry on." In our hospital, making sure that mothers on bed rest have access to books, crafts, television, and the telephone has become an integral part of the treatment. Psychopharmacology is considered when the mother is unable to sleep or becomes clinically anxious or depressed. More specific guidelines for psychotropic medications are discussed later in this chapter.

Substance abuse—Women who abuse alcohol and drugs during pregnancy are risking danger to their unborn child either by the direct effect of the substances or by the results of premature labor or low birth weight. Cocaine use can precipitate abruptio placenta. Fetal alcohol syndrome (FAS) is characterized by varying degrees of prenatal and postnatal growth retardation, dysmorphic features, and cognitive disturbances. Abrupt withdrawal from narcotics can precipitate miscarriage.

You will be frequently called to intervene with women who have a history of substance abuse. For those who are currently abstinent but fear relapse, the goal is to maximize support in the community and provide adequate treatment referrals. Regular monitoring of urine toxicology is an essential aspect of prenatal care. A woman who is on methadone maintenance for narcotic addiction should be monitored regularly by both her methadone program and her obstetrician because there may be changes in dosage requirements as the pregnancy proceeds. Symptoms of methadone withdrawal are common during the third trimester, and patients sometimes require intramuscular (IM) injections when the vomiting is severe.

For women who have failed abstinence, either by their own report or as demonstrated by clinical presentation and urine toxicology, interventions may involve outside agencies, including any current treatment programs, the legal system, the shelter system, or child protective services (CPS). In the state of New York, CPS cannot be involved until there are children in the home. A report generally has to wait until the baby is born unless there is a perceived risk to older siblings. Residential or inpatient drug treatment is still essentially voluntary unless the mother has a coexisting mental illness that is severe enough to require hospitalization. Mandated preventative services or visiting nurse services can offer some monitoring and assessment of the mother's behavior at home, but she has to be in agreement with the visits. Keep in mind that even women who have relapsed into drug use will often express concern for their babies and may even request treatment on their own to help them achieve abstinence.

Maintaining an alliance is important to promote prenatal care and ensure continuity of care (and CPS involvement, if necessary) once the baby is born.

Inadequate or noxious support systems—Pregnancy can bring couples closer together as they anticipate becoming a family. However, there are many stresses inherent to the process of reproduction, and many relationships have ended even before the arrival of the newborn. Fathers and mothers may have very different expectations, and these differences may play a key role in dealing with any complications or roadblocks. For example, one partner may view a new baby as sealing a marital bond whereas the other feels pushed away or consumed by the baby's demands. Sometimes, the father of the baby becomes overwhelmed and leaves or the relationship ends before the pregnancy was discovered. New mothers may find themselves alone or faced with reestablishing ties with a family of origin with whom they were quite ambivalent. You are often faced with the crucial task of helping a pregnant woman come to terms with how her preconceived fantasies and hopes contrast with the reality of her situation.

Domestic abuse—The incidence of domestic abuse has been found to increase during pregnancy. It has been estimated that 20% to 25% of pregnant women who seek prenatal care are victims of domestic violence. These women have increased incidence of spontaneous abortions, preterm labor, fetal injuries, and low birth weight babies. It is not uncommon for domestic violence to become evident only after a pregnant woman has been injured and requests examination. If you are called, it will be important to avoid any implication that the violence is a product of mental illness on the patient's part. There are times when an abusive partner will threaten to sue for custody on the grounds that the woman is seeing a psychiatrist and is therefore "crazy." Supportive measures often involve education and validation of the woman's experience, as well as her choices. Information about support groups, safe houses, and protective agencies can be helpful, but the woman's autonomy must be respected. She may or may not wish to make the first call to a domestic abuse hotline in your presence. There is also the sobering reality that her life may be in the most danger at the point where she makes the move to leave her partner. The vast majority of organizations for abused women are adamant that the woman is not expected to leave the relationship to seek and receive help.

When things go wrong: miscarriage, stillbirth, or impairment in a newborn—When there is a loss, the mother and her family must be given the space and opportunity to express their grief, whatever form that may take. Many hospitals now offer bereavement counseling and the obstetric wards are particularly active in reaching out to grieving patients and their families. When there is a miscarriage or death, the staff at our center offers a "memory box" that contains clothing, pictures, and any other items special to that baby or family. The couple is often encouraged to spend time alone and hold the baby or the fetus to validate and make more real the experience of their loss. You may be called to offer additional support, especially if there are concerns about postpartum depression. It is important that the experience of grief be respected and normalized for a family which may feel shaken or embarrassed by the intensity of their reactions.

Pseudocyesis—This is a relatively rare clinical state in which a woman mistakenly believes that she is pregnant and will even have some signs and symptoms of pregnancy. For example, she may have nausea, vomiting, amenorrhea, increased abdominal girth, and there have been some reports of objective changes in the breasts and cervix. The idea of pregnancy can be the only fixed delusion and there are often no hallucinations. Although this patient may not identify herself as needing psychiatric treatment, she has to be treated in a very supportive manner, especially when she is confronted with a negative pregnancy test or ultrasonography.

There is a male counterpart of this condition, called *Couvard syndrome*, in which the man actually has a type of a "pseudo-cyesis" and may gain weight during his partner's pregnancy. The man rarely will acknowledge conscious fantasies of being pregnant. He also may go through a sympathetic labor, including abdominal pain during the later phases of his wife's labor.

PSYCHIATRIC DISORDERS DURING PREGNANCY

Schizophrenia

A number of studies have documented that women with schizophrenia are at an increased risk for decompensation during and immediately after pregnancy. We also know that psychotic women are less likely to be compliant with prenatal care. Inpatient management of unstable psychotic patients results in better prenatal care but insurance usually will not cover hospitalization once the patient is stabilized.

Commonly used neuroleptics such as haloperidol, chlor-promazine, and trifluoperazine as well as the newer atypical antipsychotics such as olanzapine, risperidone, quetiapine, and ziprasidone, are rated "C" in regard to pregnancy, which means that the chance of fetal harm exists, but the clinician must weigh the risk–benefit ratio and that there are animal studies which show some harm. Interestingly, clozapine is rated "B," which means that the chance of fetal harm is remote, but possible; however, it has other potentially harmful effects that usually do not make it a first-choice drug. These ratings can change and there are essentially no definitive human research studies. Therefore, most clinicians try to avoid or minimize the dosage of any neuroleptic during the first trimester, but this may not be possible with the floridly psychotic patient. If neuroleptics are used, avoid prophylactic treatment with anticholinergic or antiparkinsonian agents because they are associated with a higher risk of malformations. If dystonic symptoms or parkinsonian side effects do occur, lower the dosage or switch to a low-potency neuroleptic medication. Also, be aware that hypocalcemia may predispose to dystonia in pregnant women who are taking neuroleptics and this can be corrected. In rare cases of neuroleptic malignant syndrome during pregnancy, bromocriptine can be used safely along with intense medical management. Although the incidence is rare, there are times when a delirious or acutely psychotic patient who is pregnant will require restraints for dangerous agitation. It is considered potentially dangerous to restrain second- and third-trimester patients in the supine (face-up) position because compression of the aorta and vena cava by the enlarged pregnant uterus may obstruct the venous blood flow to the heart and produce a hypotensive syndrome. Therefore, a pregnant patient who requires restraints should be placed on the left side, raising the right hip so that the uterus is displaced to the left. Frequent position changes should be done to prevent partial inferior vena cava obstruction and dependent edema.

Bipolar Disorder

Patients with bipolar disorder are faced with the dilemma of possible manic episodes if they go off lithium and other mood stabilizers. The use of lithium during the first trimester has been associated with cardiovascular malformations, notably Ebstein malformation (4% to 12%). More recent data has suggested that this possibility is more rare than previously thought. It can be detected by cardiac ultrasonography during pregnancy. If lithium is used, the plasma levels need to be checked because there can be increased glomerular filtration rate (GFR) in the third trimester that requires more lithium. On the contrary, at point of delivery, lowered lithium doses would be needed because of a decrease in GFR, causing increased lithium levels. In patients where a sodium restricted diet is ordered, such as women with preeclampsia and eclampsia, decreased dosage of lithium is necessary because of elevated sodium levels that result from increased reabsorption of lithium.

Valproate and carbamazepine also are considered first-line medications for bipolar disorders. However, both of them have been associated with increased incidence of neural tube defects, including *spina bifida* (1% to 2%), so they would best be avoided. This defect can be detected with special ultrasonographic techniques at 20 weeks.

We usually recommend the reinstitution of mood-stabilizing medication in a patient with bipolar illness who has just delivered because there is an increased risk of recurrence of mania or depression in the postpartum period.

Depression

The prevalence of major depression during pregnancy is 10% to 15%. The selective serotonin reuptake inhibitor (SSRI) antidepressants and other newer antidepressants are currently listed as pregnancy risk class "C," meaning that there are no human studies, but that animal studies have shown some adverse effects. However, a closer look at the current literature reveals that the animal studies used extremely high dosages and that there are increasing numbers of human studies showing little, if any, increased risk to the fetus in the first trimester. More recently, several issues have been raised: the SSRI discontinuation syndrome in the newborn, particularly with paroxetine, use of paroxetine in the first trimester, and the associated cardiovascular malformations in the newborn; the association of persistent pulmonary hypertension in the newborns of mothers who use SSRIs after 20 weeks' gestation; and the increased risk of premature delivery and lower gestational age at birth of babies born to mothers who used antidepressants during pregnancy. This has led to the label changes in SSRIs and venlafaxine with respect to their use in pregnancy. The SSRI medications have been shown to pass through the placenta barrier and to be present in breast milk. Fluoxetine, compared to the other SSRIs, has been known to cause higher infant blood levels with resulting higher adverse effects in the neonate.

When faced with the need to make clinical decisions about the use of antidepressants (or any other psychotropic medication) during pregnancy, we would suggest that you begin by doing a Medline search for recent data. It is important to remember that the risk of relapse among women who discontinue antidepressants during pregnancy is high and depression during pregnancy is one of the strongest predictors of postpartum depression. Carefully assess the patient's clinical state including potential suicidality and the potential impact on her and her family if she were to attempt to carry the pregnancy without pharmacologic treatment of her depression. This typically involves a risk–benefit analysis. In some situations, it will be quite clear that the patient needs to be on medication, but, in other cases, you and your patient may want to decide on a trial of psychotherapy without medication, especially at least through the first trimester. There clearly is a need to balance the effects of maternal use of antidepressants versus the risk of postpartum depression and the effects of avoiding psychopharmacotherapy on the mother and the baby. If you decide to use antidepressants, make sure that the mother and the father both give informed consent and document this. Electroconvulsive therapy (ECT) has been used during pregnancy without adverse effects and avoids the risk of medications. In the late stages of pregnancy, we recommend having an obstetric consultant in a standby mode during the administration of ECT.

Anxiety and the Use of Sedative Hypnotics

Some women become very anxious in anticipation of pregnancy or during pregnancy.

Benzodiazepines are not recommended for continuous use during the first trimester. However, they may play a role, if sparingly used, during the second or third trimester for women who have severe panic episodes or are under major stress, such as those undergoing strict bed rest on tocolytics. In these cases, both mother and baby should be monitored to prevent overly sedating the baby (as evidenced by diminished reactivity or movement). When used in larger doses during the later phases, especially during labor, there is the possibility of "floppy baby syndrome," which includes hypotonia, lethargy, and sucking difficulties. There also can be a withdrawal syndrome that would include tremors, irritability, and hypertonicity. Benzodiazepines also are not recommended during breastfeeding.

Human Immunodeficiency Virus Disease

The number of women who are infected with human immuno-deficiency virus (HIV) is increasing and most of these women are of childbearing age. In the United States, it is estimated that between 1 and 2 of every 1,000 women who give birth are HIV infected, approximately 5,000 to 7,000 women annually. Advances in the care and treatment of the pregnant woman with HIV, particularly using effective combination antiretro-viral therapy have decreased perinatal transmission rate to 1% to 2%. Most transmission, approximately two-thirds, occurs late in pregnancy or at the time of delivery by transvaginal or transplacental exposure. Because of this, the benefit of prenatal counseling in reducing high-risk sexual behaviors as well as encouraging women to test for HIV as early as possible cannot be overemphasized.

Current combination treatment for HIV has resulted in improved prognosis with HIV patients now living longer. This has led to more women and men with HIV with a desire to have children of their own. There are certain issues that need to be recognized in this special population. First, simply contem-plating pregnancy will be fraught with psychological conflicts (i.e., "I want to have a baby so much, but how can I morally risk the exposure to HIV?"). Second, there are the risks and benefits of being on antiretroviral therapy, including potential problems with fetal development. On the whole, there are sev-eral opportunities for you, as a C-L psychiatrist, to intervene in the psychological care of the HIV-infected woman.

ELECTIVE ABORTION

Emotions often run high when the issue of elective abor-tion comes up. Even when abortion is chosen, some loss is experienced by the woman and there is usually some kind of grieving, which may or may not be short-lived. Women who have decided to terminate an unwanted pregnancy may describe a mixture of relief and loss, as they come to terms with previous fantasies about pregnancy and children. They also sometimes report a fear or a sense of loss regarding their bodily integrity. Those who have terminated a pregnancy because of a medical catastrophe (e.g., certain life-threatening conditions in the mother or multiple congenital anomalies in the fetus) tend to grieve for the lost child in a similar manner as those who have miscarried. Sometimes the situation is complicated by other factors such as the conflicting reactions of family and staff. For example, staff may express concern and empathy for the mother, while, at the same time, struggling with their own personal feelings about pregnancy and childbirth. When the family is involved, the patient must deal with their reactions and values as well as her own at a time when she may feel quite vulnerable.

CASE VIGNETTE: ABORTION IN A JEHOVAH'S WITNESS

A 16-year-old Jehovah's Witness unmarried female, living with her parents, who had one child (aged 2) was sure that she would never let herself become involved in a situation where she would become pregnant again. She was embarking upon a new career and a life as a single mother. When she ultimately realized that she had become pregnant by her boyfriend, she approached various medical agencies for an abortion. She found herself unable to afford the medical fees and became frightened that she might not be able to have the abortion. She then tried to induce an abortion with a pair of scissors. She was admitted with a critically low hemoglobin from bleeding. Her parents, and initially the patient, prohibited any blood transfusion based on religious belief. The patient continued to request an abortion. Finally, after much exploration with the psychiatrist and other health care providers, she made a private agreement with the hospital that she would accept transfusion, but only if her life was in immediate danger. She then underwent an elective abortion, which was completed without a transfusion. The C-L psychiatrist had numerous meetings with the patient, family, and the treatment staff. Intense emotions were generated in various staff members, which needed to be addressed, as did the emotional state of the patient and family.

POSTPARTUM "BLUES"

Most new mothers (estimated 50% to 80%) will have mood swings, usually beginning 3 to 4 days after delivery. During these times, the woman may feel anxious, irritable, or tearful, with difficulty sleeping. Postpartum blues may be interspersed with periods of feeling well. The symptoms may worsen during the later part of the first week and will usually mostly resolve by the end of the second week after delivery. It is when these symptoms last more than 2 weeks or when there are any hallmarks of major depression or any suggestions of suicidal or homicidal ideation that immediate psychiatric attention and follow-up is required.

POSTPARTUM DEPRESSION

The risk factors for postpartum depression are previous pregnancy-related depressive episodes (50% to 60%), previous history of major depression (approximately 30%), previous history of bipolar disorder (33% to 50%), family history of depression, poor social support, adverse life events, marital instability, and ambivalence toward the pregnancy.

According to Diagnostic and Statistical Manual of Mental Disorders, Fourth Edition (DSM-IV) criteria, a depressive episode qualifies as postpartum depression when it occurs within the first 4 weeks of delivery. Although hormonal changes, exhaustion after delivery, sleep deprivation due to caring for the baby, as well as emotional stress, may contribute to the symptoms that the patient is having, you should not minimize depressive symptoms in the postpartum period. It is estimated that between 12% and 16% of all women experience a postpartum depressive episode, and the percentage is almost twice that for adolescent mothers. Pay close attention to any feelings of guilt that the mother may have, as well as fears about being a "bad mother." Similarly, when there are concerns that some harm will come to the baby (that go beyond normal worries that a new mother may have), it is a good clue that you are dealing with an insidious postpartum depression. Sometimes, rather than insomnia, there may be hypersomnia and, rather than poor appetite, the patient may show hyperphagia, particularly when there is a bipolar condition.

As with any other patient, suicidal or homicidal ideation in this setting should be taken seriously. There is a dual risk to mother and infant if symptoms occur and it does not make sense to wait for some criteria threshold to be reached when there are concerns about this condition. The existence of a support system and the presence of someone to observe the mother with the baby and assist or take over the care, when necessary, should be taken into account in these situations.

Treatment of Postpartum Depression

Individual assessment of the patient will best determine the type and extent of treatment. As noted in the more mild forms of postpartum blues, support and monitoring may be all that is required. Extra help in caring for the newborn may be very valuable in all forms of these conditions. Antidepressant treatment with psychotherapy may be the treatment of choice. SSRI medication combined with mood stabilizer may be indicated in bipolar disorder. (See the following text for a discussion of considerations when the mother is nursing.) In the more severe forms of postpartum mood disorder or when there is a danger to the patient or baby, hospitalization usually is indicated and sometimes ECT may be a useful treatment modality. Aggressive treatment of postpartum depression will limit the incapacity of the mother and also may reduce the possibility of diminished mother–infant bonding and attachment, which may affect the long-term emotional development of the newborn.

POSTPARTUM PSYCHOSIS

Postpartum psychosis usually will develop within the first 2 weeks, if it is going to occur, and can occur as early as 48 hours. It occurs in approximately 1 or 2 per 1,000 postpartum women and needs to be recognized immediately because of its tendency to rapidly escalate. Early symptoms of restlessness, irritability, and insomnia escalate rapidly to depressed or manic mood, disorganized behavior, labile mood, hallucinations, or delusions. The presentation may be that of a manic episode, which then will progress to overt psychosis, often with delirium-like symptoms and confusion. Hospitalization usually is needed in any case of postpartum psychosis because of the risk of suicide or infanticide. Once there has been a postpartum psychosis, the chances of it occurring during a second pregnancy, without prophylactic treatment, is estimated to be as great as 75% to 90%.

*CASE VIGNETTE: WHEN BLUES PROGRESS
TO POSTPARTUM DEPRESSION AND INFANTICIDE*

*The patient was a married 33-year-old mother of a 2-year-old
child who just delivered her second child. The patient had a
history of being treated for major depression when she was in
her early twenties, but she had had no treatment since that
time. Immediately after delivery from an uneventful pregnancy,
the patient felt "quite blue," which progressed over the next
month. At first, she was not enthusiastic about her new child
although she took care of him in a satisfactory manner and
was successfully nursing. She then became increasingly fearful
that something would happen to her children. She became
religiously preoccupied, which she had not been in the past.
She became very fearful that the devil would kill her children.
While her paranoid ideas were of concern to her family, they
believed that she was improving. She was taking care of the
children, but she became delusionally preoccupied and believed
that the only way she could save her children from the devil
was to kill them and then join them by killing herself. She
smothered and killed both of her children and then swallowed
lye in an attempt to kill herself.*

*When seen in psychiatric consultation, she was in a catatonic
state. With some difficulty, it was possible to elicit the fact that
she was having command hallucinations, which made her kill
her children and attempt to take her own life. She also had
paranoid ideas that people and the devil wanted to hurt her.
She was treated with haloperidol (5 mg twice a day by mouth).
Within 3 days, her delusions and hallucinations went into
remission. At this point, she became profoundly depressed. She
curled into the fetal position and was tearful most of the time.
She ate very little, slept poorly, and would not talk about her
children. Otherwise, her speech, while not spontaneous, was
relevant and coherent and did not have psychotic content or
evidence of a thought disorder. She would not deny that she
felt suicidal.*

*The patient was then treated with fluoxetine (20 mg), which
was increased to 40 mg per day. After 2.5 weeks, she appeared
to be less anxious, began to show hunger, and slept with a
more normal pattern. She was still quite sad and would not talk
about her children and would become tearful whenever they
were mentioned. She also would not respond to questions about
her suicidality. The patient was lost to follow-up when she was
transferred to a forensic unit of a correctional institution.*

LIAISON POTENTIAL

There is often special interest on the part of obstetricians in having a psychiatric consultant who specializes in the psychological issues that are related to pregnancy. Such a person (most likely a female psychiatrist) would be very attuned to all the stresses related to the different stages of pregnancy, as well as being up-to-date on the use of psychotropic medications during pregnancy and breastfeeding. This person might make regular rounds on the obstetric unit and attend special case conferences. She also could participate in various specialized activities (listed in subsequent text), although it is also likely that a psychiatrist might be dedicated to any one of the following liaison activities.

1. Special consultant to a high-risk obstetric unit where patients are hospitalized for various conditions threatening the pregnancy.
2. Consultant to women who have had perinatal loss. This also involves running groups and working with nurses and other staff who often find this a very difficult area in which to work.
3. Consultant to a fertility clinic. The complicated new techniques bring with them many psychological stresses on both the woman and her partner.
4. Consultant to a birth control/abortion clinic. This involves many challenges, which often includes substance abuse and adolescents as well as people from all walks of life.

Psychiatric Aspects of Women's Health

There has been increasing evidence in the literature about the important relationship between reproductive endocrinology and mental health in women. Psychiatric disorders have been shown to be affected by changes in the gonadal hormones and neurotransmitters. It has been observed that there are exacerbations of psychiatric disorders in women in the premenstrual, postpartum, and perimenopausal periods of their lives. New-onset psychiatric disorders in pregnancy as well as during the menstrual cycles suggest a role for estrogen and progesterone in the expression of affective and psychotic disorders in women. In this chapter we will be focusing on psychological issues throughout a woman's menstrual cycle as well as specific issues associated with women's health such as infertility, cancer, domestic violence and abuse, substance abuse, and cardiovascular disease. We will also briefly address the difference between women and men in the prevalence, course, and response to treatment of some psychiatric disorders. Pregnancy is addressed in a separate chapter, whereas eating disorders are addressed in Chapter 8. Although some of the topics here are also briefly addressed in other chapters, we believe that some points need to be reinforced if only to stress their importance.

DISORDERS RELATED TO THE MENSTRUAL CYCLE

Premenstrual Syndrome

Premenstrual syndrome or PMS, as it is more commonly called, is a group of mood, behavioral, and/or physical symptoms that occur during the luteal phase of most menstrual cycles. Emotional symptoms include depression, anxiety, irritability, mood swings, and anger. Behavioral symptoms include sleep disorders, food cravings, and increased appetite. Physical symptoms include bloating, breast tenderness, headaches, and joint and muscle pains. The symptoms must remit once the menstrual flow ends and there is a symptom-free interval for about a week or more each cycle. There has been evidence to suggest that women with PMS have an increased risk of developing major depression in their lifetime. Treatment of PMS is usually supportive: lifestyle changes (decreased stress, exercise, relaxation techniques), dietary measures (avoid caffeine), and sleep hygiene.

All other agents, including vitamins, calcium, and diuretics, have not been consistently effective. There have been more recent studies, however, that indicate that estrogen may be beneficial but more placebo-controlled double-blind studies need to be done.

Premenstrual Dysphoric Disorder

Like PMS, PMDD also has a cyclic relationship to the luteal phase of the menstrual cycle. According to Diagnostic and Statistical Manual of Mental Disorders, Fourth Edition, Text Revision (DSM-IV-TR), to make the diagnosis there has to be a minimum of 5 out of 11 symptoms, one of which must be a mood symptom (Table 7.1). In addition, the symptoms must interfere with work, school, and/or relationships, and be confirmed by charting symptoms daily for two cycles. This must not be an exacerbation of another disorder.

TABLE 7.1. Symptom Criteria for Premenstrual
Dysphoric Disorder (PMDD)

Depression	Fatigue
Anxiety	Change in appetite
Mood swings	Sleep disturbances
Irritability	Feeling overwhelmed
Decreased interest	Other physical symptoms such
Difficulty concentrating	as bloating, breast tenderness

(Data from American Psychiatric Association. *Diagnostic and statistical manual of mental disorders*, 4th ed. Text revised. Washington, DC: American Psychiatric Association, 2000:771–774.)

Current research has shown that selective serotonin reuptake inhibitors (SSRIs) and serotonin norepinephrine reuptake inhibitors (SNRIs) are effective in treating the affective, behavioral, and physical symptoms of PMDD. More recently, intermittent dosing (taking medications only during the luteal phase) was also found to be effective so this will appeal to women who do not want to take medication daily.

CASE VIGNETTE: "THE WOMAN WHO COULD NOT UNDERSTAND"

A 35-year-old woman presented to a psychiatrist in a Women's Clinic. She complained of lability, depression, and irritability, which usually occur about a day before her menstrual period begins. At the same time, she observed that she felt bloated and fatigued and had no appetite. She stated she would cry unabashedly at the slightest thing and could not understand why. She initially did not relate it to her menstrual cycle until she noted this happened every month. She began recording her menstrual cycle and mood changes as requested by her psychiatrist. She was started on effexor (Venlafaxine) and after a month, she began feeling better.

Menopause

The hormonal changes that occur during menopause (mainly decreased estrogen and progesterone levels) are associated with vasomotor episodes known as *hot flashes* and may cause anxiety, distress, and insomnia. In some women, there is significant psychological meaning in having reached this stage of the reproductive cycle that can lead to feelings of loss and depression. There have been studies that show that women are at an increased risk for depression during the perimenopausal period. Perimenopause is the period that starts during the early menopausal transition until the woman has amenorrhea for 12 months. Although it is not clearly established, some clinicians and researchers believe that perimenopausal depression is a distinct entity that may or may not be due directly to the hormonal changes.

The decision to utilize hormonal replacement therapy (HRT) is complex and somewhat controversial. It should be based on the latest evidence-based research, as well as the risk factors that the patient may have for cardiovascular disease and various types of cancer. In addition, the use of SSRIs and other antidepressants should be considered in the treatment of menopausal women with clinically significant depressive symptoms. Recent studies have shown that postmenopausal women with depression and vasomotor symptoms show significant improvement in depression, vasomotor symptoms, sleep, anxiety, and pain after SSRI treatment. If there are significant psychological issues around this phase of life, various forms of psychotherapy, including insight and cognitive-oriented therapies, can be effective with or without psychopharmacotherapy.

As a consultation-liaison (C-L) psychiatrist, you may encounter patients with menstrual cycle–related disorders during the course of evaluating women in the general hospital setting or in women's outpatient clinics, such as gynecology clinics. It is important to keep PMS and PMDD in the differential when evaluating females for depression.

INFERTILITY

Infertility is defined as the inability to conceive after a year of sexual intercourse without contraception. While both men and women can be infertile, in the past, women who were infertile were associated with some form of psychopathology. There has been less emphasis on this as infertility treatments have become available. Among causes of infertility are disorders of ovulation, semen abnormalities, damaged tubes, depression, and eating disorders. There are medications that may cause psychiatric symptoms such as depression, mood swings, even psychosis. Drug–drug interactions need to be also considered. If medications do not work, assisted reproductive technology is the other option. This includes *in vitro* fertilization, intracytoplasmic sperm injection, and third party parenting (traditional surrogate or gestational surrogate).

There are ethical concerns as well as emotional issues that can complicate the situation where a C-L psychiatrist can play a role. You may also be helpful in supporting the multidisciplinary staff of a fertility team who may find the work emotionally draining due to failure of pregnancy, ethical, and legal issues.

CASE VIGNETTE: "THE WOMAN IN THE ER"

A 50-year-old woman presents herself to the emergency room (ER), complaining of pain in the arms and back as well as shortness of breath. Electrocardiogram (ECG) and chest x-ray were within normal limits. The ER physician requested a psychiatry consult for anxiety. The patient was seen and evaluated. Although anxious because of her current condition, the patient did not have a previous history of anxiety. By the time the evaluation was completed, the cardiac enzymes came back elevated. The patient was treated for an acute myocardial event.

HEART DISEASE

Women with cardiac disease are different from men in many ways. Some of the risk factors such as obesity, diabetes, and smoking (especially when on oral contraceptives) cause more risk in women than in men. Elevated triglycerides and low high-density lipoprotein (HDL) have also greater risk in women than in men. In terms of presentation, women more often complain of atypical pain, and are more likely to have shortness of breath, palpitations, fatigue, and nausea than men. Women may also not have Q waves in their ECG during a myocardial infarction (MI). In terms of treatment, women are less likely to receive medications that men receive or be recommended for cardiac catheterization as men are. The prognosis for women with cardiac disease is also worse than that of men. This is because women are older and have more complications such as diabetes, hypertension, or hyperlipidemia. Physicians are also less aggressive in diagnosing and treating women with cardiac disorders. Attribution of symptoms to anxiety, depression, and somatization often interfere with the diagnosis.

However, more studies are needed to examine why this is so. As a C-L psychiatrist, you will likely be asked to see these patients in the ER or in the hospital unit so it is important to make sure the diagnosis of an actual cardiac event is not missed.

WOMEN AND CANCER

Gynecologic cancers were briefly addressed in Chapter 3. In this chapter we would like to specifically address the different kinds of gynecologic cancers.

Endometrial Cancer

The most common risk factor for this cancer is exposure to estrogen. It is of interest to note that most (70%) women with endometrial cancer are postmenopausal. Although women with this type of cancer have a better prognosis, there are still significant psychological issues that face women with endometrial cancer. The loss of the uterus, which is the symbol of their identity as a woman, may affect the woman's sense of self. Sexual dysfunction is a complication, which may be not only physiological but also psychological in origin.

Cervical Cancer

Although the mortality of this type of cancer has been significantly reduced with the increased numbers of women having annual screenings with the Papanicolau test (Pap screen), there are still women, particularly those who have had sexual trauma, who absolutely refuse to have the test. It is not only their fear of having cancer but the memories/flashbacks that may be precipitated by the procedure that is preventing them from taking the test. As with the other forms of gynecologic cancers, body image, sexuality, and self-esteem are psychological concerns in this group. In addition, because this cancer affects more childbearing women, they wrestle with the possibility of losing their ability to have children. The various treatment modalities: chemotherapy, surgery, and radiation therapy all come with side effects that lead to sexual dysfunction that, for some, continue to occur 5 years after treatment.

Ovarian Cancer

Of all the gynecologic cancers, ovarian cancer is the leading cause of death. The problem with ovarian cancer is that there are no early symptoms or screening test to alert us to the presence of this disease. By the time it is diagnosed, the disease is already in the advanced stages. Because of this, the women with ovarian cancer have a higher level of distress when compared to other cancers. In addition to the expected mortality, women with ovarian cancer frequently have recurrences and complications. Similar to the other gynecologic cancers, women with ovarian cancer often experience sexual dysfunction with treatment.

Breast Cancer

With increased mammography screenings and advances in research and treatment, more and more women survive breast cancer now more than ever. Breast reconstruction with implants that are done immediately after the surgery helps in coping with the self-esteem and body image issues that women undergoing radical bilateral mastectomies often experience. With the emergence of genetic testing, women with a family history of breast cancer will in some instances opt for a bilateral mastectomy with reconstruction even if they do not have any evidence of the presence of breast cancer. One of the important steps in the preoperative clearance of patients who undergo prophylactic mastectomy is a psychiatric clearance that C-L psychiatrists often are asked to do.

DOMESTIC VIOLENCE

Although domestic violence has been briefly addressed in Chapter 6, you may also come across this issue in the medical–surgical units and in the ER. Domestic violence involves assaultive or coercive behavior against an intimate partner, which may be physical, sexual, economic, and psychological threats or attacks. Victims of domestic violence often do not disclose that information either because they are afraid of additional violence or because they are embarrassed about it. You may be asked to determine whether domestic violence exists or when they suspect that this may be present, you may be asked to intervene. Certain signs should alert you to the possibility that the patient is a victim: injuries are not consistent with the reported cause, there are multiple injuries in various stages of healing, any injury in pregnant women, and evasiveness about how an injury occurred. The presence of anxiety, depression, suicidality, alcohol/drug abuse, and the presence of a partner who seems overly concerned or controlling are also warning signs of the possibility of domestic violence. Your primary concern should be the safety of the patient. This should be accompanied by a multidisciplinary approach, which is based on confidentiality, communication, and coordination. Referrals to shelters or alternative living situations and legal motions such as order of protection, counseling, and advocates for domestic violence are very important.

You should not forget to give the number of the National Domestic Violence Hotline (1-800-799-SAFE).

CASE VIGNETTE: "PERSISTENCE IN DIAGNOSING DOMESTIC ABUSE"

A 25-year-old woman was admitted for surgical repair of her fractured right humerus. The surgeon noted that the patient's explanation for the fracture did not appear to explain the injury and he suspected domestic violence. He asked the psychiatrist to see the patient. The patient was lying in the hospital bed with a cast and her husband was seated next to her. He refused to leave to allow the psychiatrist to see the patient alone and the patient told the psychiatrist that she wants him in the room during the interview. The psychiatrist briefly saw the patient and left. She returned later after visiting hours and after a long discussion, the patient admitted to the abuse. The psychiatrist then started the process of keeping the patient safe and getting the social worker to arrange for alternative living situation on discharge.

SUBSTANCE ABUSE IN WOMEN

Women are much less likely to report substance abuse than men. This could be due to social stigma and stereotyping. Women who abuse alcohol and other substances frequently report gastric problems, insomnia, and other physical symptoms. They likely present with depression and anxiety and use the substances to cope with these issues.

However, women, when compared to men, can be more sensitive to the toxic effects of alcohol and other substances (i.e., they experience a more toxic effect from the same dose as men) and can develop dependence more easily than men. Because women are less likely to volunteer information on substance use, it is important to ask the questions in a nonconfrontational manner. Across the lifespan, women may vary as to their risk factors for alcohol and substance use. In their 20s and 30s, they may combine alcohol with illicit drug use and engage in binge drinking. Middle-aged women often drink at home when they are alone and may abuse prescribed psychoactive drugs or combine alcohol and tranquilizers, whereas older women are more likely to abuse prescription drugs than alcohol.

PSYCHIATRIC DISORDERS: THE GENDER DIFFERENCE

Women are much more likely than men to meet criteria for different anxiety disorders in their lifetime. There have been significant gender differences in the onset and clinical course of anxiety disorders. There is a difference in the manifestation of bipolar disorder in women versus men. Women are more likely to have a later age of onset and the seasonal pattern is more common in women. Women also experience more depressive episodes and are more likely to have rapid cycling. Substance use disorders are more common in men, whereas medical comorbidity, anxiety, and eating disorders are more common in women.

However, there is no notable gender difference in treatment response between men and women but women are more likely to experience side effects such as weight gain and hypothyroidism with lithium and polycystic ovary syndrome with valproic acid.

Psychiatric Aspects of Women's Health 97

LIAISON OPPORTUNITIES

1. Work as a psychiatrist colocated in a Women's Clinic.
2. Participate as a member of a multidisciplinary fertility team.
3. Be the psychiatric liaison in a Gynecology Clinic or inpatient treatment team.
4. Be a psychiatric liaison in a breast cancer clinic or inpatient treatment team.
5. Start a support group for women with cancer in a unit/clinic.

Psychiatric Aspects of Gastroenterology

Essential Concepts

- Multiple factors contribute to peptic ulcer, rather than a specific personality state.
- Difficulty in swallowing, with a lump in the throat, is typical of anxiety symptoms, although there are other possible causes.
- Patients with irritable bowel syndrome (IBS) usually have abnormal motility and a histologically normal colon that is often influenced by psychological factors.
- Patients with inflammatory bowel disorder (IBD) have diagnosable inflammatory lesions in the gastrointestinal (GI) tract that can require intensive medical/surgical treatment and can have psychiatric comorbidity.
- Pancreatic cancer can present with depression and anxiety before diagnosis.
- The mortality rates of eating disorders can be as high as 15% to 20%.
- Patients with anorexia nervosa have an intense fear of gaining weight or being fat, although they may be quite underweight.
- Patients with bulimia nervosa often will engage in compensatory behavior for their binging by purging themselves or by using enemas, laxatives, or excessive exercises, all of which could be harmful to their health.

The gut and its relationship to emotions have been a focus of interest since the early years of psychosomatic medicine. Some of the most fascinating research in psychosomatic medicine was done with patients who had gastric fistulas. Fistulas allow direct visualization of parts of the GI tract. Both gastric resection and motility have been shown to be influenced by the emotional state of the patient.

In this chapter, we focus on a variety of clinical situations that you are likely to encounter among hospitalized patients, each of which involves the gut. In some cases, GI pathology causes psychological distress (as in inflammatory bowel disease); in other cases, a psychiatric problem causes the GI disturbance (as in eating disorders). In still other situations, the relationship between mind and gut is likely a two-way street (as in peptic ulcer and IBS).

PEPTIC ULCER

While early psychoanalytic theory suggested a connection between peptic ulcer and dependency conflicts, we now know that the bacteria, *Helicobacter pylori*, is a primary cause of peptic ulcers and other gastric erosions. Nonetheless, a number of psychologically mediated factors, such as alcohol and tobacco use, also are associated with erosive lesions. In addition, extreme psychophysiological stress, poor social support, and an inability to express emotions (known as *alexithymia*) have all been identified as potential risk factors for the development of gastric and duodenal lesions. You also should be aware that some of the medications used to treat peptic ulcer, especially the H_2-receptor antagonists, such as cimetidine, ranitidine, and famotidine, may cause delirium and/or depression.

FUNCTIONAL DYSPEPSIA

Primary care physicians often will refer patients to you with a diagnosis of "functional (nonulcer) dyspepsia," which is characterized by recurrent upper abdominal pain for at least 3 months with no objective evidence of any lesions. Such nonorganic dyspepsia may be symptomatic of depression, anxiety disorders, or, more rarely, psychotic disorders.

SWALLOWING DIFFICULTIES AND ESOPHAGEAL DYSFUNCTION

You frequently will be in a position to evaluate a patient who is complaining of some difficulty in swallowing where it has been determined that there is no organic lesion. The typical complaint is that there is a "lump in my throat." This symptom, referred to as *globus hystericus* in the earlier psychoanalytic literature, is often a feature of somatization disorder or panic disorder and can be effectively treated with antianxiety medication or psychotherapy.

IRRITABLE BOWEL SYNDROME

Patients with IBS present with changes in their bowel habits, with or without abdominal pain. IBS is primarily a disorder of bowel motility and such patients have histologically normal colons. Although IBS may have an organic basis, the prevalence and incidence of IBS are strongly associated with the presence of stress. There is also evidence of central alpha-adrenergic receptor dysfunction in this condition. Therefore, it is not surprising that various studies have suggested that psychological stress worsens irritable bowel symptoms. Patients with IBS who seek treatment have been found to have a higher rate of certain psychiatric conditions, such as anxiety or depressive disorders. Many patients can cite a stressful event preceding the onset of their symptoms. It is noteworthy that these patients often have greater psychological impairment than patients with IBD as described in the subsequent text.

INFLAMMATORY BOWEL DISORDER

Regional enteritis, known as *Crohn's disease (CD)*, which involves the small bowel, and ulcerative colitis (UC), which involves the colon, make up the entity known as *IBD*.

In contrast to IBS, the two disorders listed under IBD have diagnosable inflammatory lesions in the GI tract. These patients can develop marked abnormalities in fluid and electrolyte balance as a result of their diarrhea. Loss of blood and malabsorption of nutrients also can lead to anemia. Patients with IBD often require stressful treatments that could include multiple surgeries, colostomies, steroid treatment, and artificial nutrition. These conditions can cause delirium. As a result of the effects of the disease and its treatment, patients with IBD can have significant psychological symptoms and impaired social functioning. The full range of symptoms related to steroids, which include steroid psychosis, delirium, and depression, can be seen. In addition, these patients also can have comorbid psychiatric disorders, which may or may not be related to IBD. These comorbid psychiatric disorders, particularly when they involve pain or other somatization symptoms, may alter the perception of the severity of the disease in some patients. This could lead to unnecessary aggressive treatments.

There is some suggestion in the literature that there are differences in personality between patients with CD and those with UC. It appears that patients with CD are more likely to have lifetime psychiatric disorders than are patients with UC. This association is more modest than those with IBS.

LIVER DISEASE

As a consultation-liaison (C-L) psychiatrist, you should always make good eye contact with patients. Therefore, icteric sclera should not be missed and, occasionally, psychiatrists are the first to pick up the presence of liver disease.

Liver disease can affect psychological functioning in many ways, both directly and indirectly. Many of the complications of liver disease, such as myopathy, fractures, diarrhea, incontinence, hypoglycemia, and others, lead to significant psychiatric morbidity, such as depression and anxiety. Also consider the effects of liver disease on sexual function and sleep patterns. Patients with liver disease also can have problems tolerating psychotropic medications.

Liver Transplantation

In recent years, liver transplantation has become more common for patients with alcoholic liver disease as well as other causes and has many psychiatric considerations. There is some disagreement as to whether liver transplantation should be offered to alcoholics who have not had a significant period of abstinence. Before a transplant, you may be asked to see patients to evaluate whether a psychiatric contraindication to the transplant exists. You should evaluate the chances of alcohol relapse, the quality of the patient's social support network, any active substance use, and history of adherence to treatment recommendations. Although the presence of psychiatric disorders does not automatically disqualify a person for liver transplantation, it is important to be able to evaluate the current state of the patient's psychiatric disorder. Partial liver transplantation is now available from live donors, which brings with it the usual psychological issues related to organ donation. In addition, remember that neuropsychiatric syndromes, especially delirium and neurotoxic effects of antirejection drugs, are common in transplant patients.

Hepatitis

Screening for hepatitis is routine during most hospitalizations. Hepatitis C often is associated with intravenous (IV) substance abuse or sexual transmission, whereas hepatitis A is contracted by the fecal–oral route, usually by eating contaminated food. Patients with the latter may be wrongly assumed to be substance abusers, which can create additional psychological stress. Because either form can progress to life-threatening illness, often in relatively young people, the possibility of a liver transplant becomes a consideration here. Hepatitis also should be considered in the differential diagnosis of patients who present with persistent fatigue, which may include patients who are thought to have depression. Hepatitis C infection progresses very slowly, so that often after being asymptomatic for 20 years or more, patients are now being told their livers are failing. There were an estimated 4.1 million Americans with hepatitis C as of 2004 with 26,000 new infections per year. It is important to note that in the treatment of hepatitis C, peginterferon and ribavirin causes depression, suicidality, irritability, and even mania. Oftentimes, before the infectious disease (ID) specialists or GI specialists start interferon, a psychiatric clearance is requested for patients who have a psychiatric history. This does not mean that patients with a psychiatric history are not eligible for treatment, but they should be regularly monitored for the possibility of the emergence of psychiatric side effects.

Acute Intermittent Porphyria

Acute intermittent porphyria (AIP) is an autosomal dominant condition that is caused by a genetic defect of the deaminase gene, which is located on chromosome 11. This results in porphobilinogen accumulation and storage. The diagnosis is made by detecting an excess of porphobilinogen in the urine during the acute episode. Interepisode tests may be inconclusive. Typical symptoms consist of acute abdominal pain, vomiting, severe constipation, pain in the back and legs, seizures, and status epilepticus, as well as motor peripheral neuropathy with weakness, numbness, and paresthesisas. This can progress to Guillain-Barre syndrome. Delirium is the most common neuropsychiatric manifestation. The full range of other psychiatric symptoms includes depression and other psychotic manifestations. This is a rare illness, but it belongs in the differential diagnosis of abdominal pain. Because the diagnosis is often missed in an initial workup, you may have an opportunity to make it while evaluating patients for so-called functional pain.

Wilson's Disease

Wilson's disease is a rare autosomal recessive disorder of copper transport, which presents with neuropsychiatric and hepatic symptoms. Patients can have abdominal pain, tremors, dystonia, ataxia, hepatic disease, hemolytic anemia, and Kayser-Fleisher ring in the eyes, as well as personality changes, psychotic manifestations, and dementia. Although rare, it should be part of the differential diagnosis in patients who present at initial onset with psychiatric symptoms and liver disease. Treatment involves utilizing chelating agents for copper toxicity, while psychiatric symptoms are treated symptomatically.

PANCREATIC CANCER

Cancer of the pancreas is frequently fatal, and less than one-third of patients with this type of cancer have an operable condition. It also appears that people with this condition will often present with depression and anxiety before the condition is diagnosed. Because of the poor prognosis and the debilitating nature of the illness, patients frequently will become very depressed once they find out that they have this illness. Individual short-term therapy, usually supportive type or group therapy techniques, can be offered to patients with any cancer and can be particularly helpful to the patient who is overwhelmed with a diagnosis of pancreatic cancer.

EATING DISORDERS

The treatment of various eating disorders usually takes place in specialized units, often with specialized techniques. However, you usually will be called to help diagnose such patients in the medical/surgical setting, which can be difficult because the patient may deny or minimize his or her abnormal eating pattern. This is a serious task because some long-term studies have reported mortality rates as high as 15% to 20%. A brief review of the various types of common eating disorders follows.

Anorexia nervosa—Most commonly found in young women (usually having onset in early teenage years), with prevalence conservatively estimated as between 0.3% and 0.8%. This condition, characterized by a refusal to maintain body weight at or above a minimally normal weight for age and height, is defined as a body weight of less than 85% of expected weight. The patient often expresses an intense fear of gaining weight or becoming fat, although she may be quite underweight. Not infrequently, the facial appearance will not give away the very thin, sometimes emaciated, appearance of the other parts of the body, which the patient will attempt to conceal. Menstrual periods characteristically will have stopped and the patient will have little concern about this situation. A history of the abnormal eating pattern from the family may be helpful in making the diagnosis. In the restrictive type of anorexia nervosa, weight loss is achieved through severe dieting alone, whereas in the binge eating/purging type, the patient regularly engages in binge eating or purging behavior, such as self-induced vomiting or the misuse of laxatives, diuretics, or enemas.

Bulimia nervosa—This type of eating disorder has an estimated prevalence of approximately 1% to 5%. It is also much more common in females and has an onset in adolescence or early adulthood. It is characterized by eating a greater than normal amount of food in a 2-hour period and feeling out of control during this episode. There is also inappropriate compensatory behavior, such as self-induced vomiting; misuse of laxatives, diuretics, or other medications; enemas, or excessive exercise.

Both of these conditions may be much more prevalent than noted earlier and may actually exist in a subclinical state or may not come to the attention of psychiatrists unless the patient is hospitalized for another condition and concern is raised about the patient's weight or eating pattern. You should be alert for this condition in persons who might be under unusual pressure to diet, such as actresses, models, dancers, and perhaps any young woman where there would be psychodynamics leading her in this direction. There is high comorbidity with depression, substance abuse disorders, and a variety of personality disorders.

Chronic vomiting can cause serious dental problems, whereas any purging behavior can lead to electrolyte imbalances that can be life threatening. Malnourishment also can be fatal and it is possible to starve to death if appropriate interventions are not made. You may end up using a form of behavioral therapy that would involve negotiating with the patient to achieve a certain weight to terminate the IV or parental treatment and ultimately discharge from the medical hospitalization. This is obviously a quick fix, which will not change the underlying problems that led to the hospitalization. The main goal will be for the patient to accept a long-term specialized treatment program that can be on an inpatient or outpatient basis.

CASE VIGNETTE: HIDDEN EATING DISORDER

The patient was a 32-year-old woman who was admitted to the neurology service for a severe migraine and protracted vomiting. After receiving IV fluids and medication for the migraine, her symptoms were mostly improved, but it was felt that she was quite depressed and was noted to have decreased appetite, with approximately a 5- to 10-lb weight loss over the previous 3 months. The patient acknowledged depressed feelings about a recent breakup with her boyfriend 4 months previously. She had been in psychotherapy with a social worker on and off for the last 5 years and denied ever being suicidal. Because of the depression, on the day of the planned discharge, a psychiatric consultation was requested.

On entering the patient's room, the patient was eating and she pushed away a full tray of food and noted that she was finished. She sipped a large bottle of water throughout the interview. The patient was complaining of a hematoma at the site of an IV that had recently been removed. The consultant took that opportunity to look at it and check for tenderness, which it was not. However, it was very clear that her arms were extremely thin compared to her normal-appearing face. She was 5 ft 2 in. tall and her weight was recorded as 100 lb. There actually were some small cuts on her left hand by the knuckles, not unlike that reported to be present in women who induce vomiting. The patient denied any eating problems and stated, if anything, she thought she was too heavy. She also reported that she vigorously exercised a few hours per night and was a runner. She shared her history of a very tumultuous dysfunctional family and her own history of having numerous failed relationships.

The patient indicated that she was ready to find a new psychotherapist and she was referred to the outpatient therapist who was experienced in working with eating disorders, which was what the patient was believed to have. The diagnosis of anorexia nervosa with purging and binge eating was confirmed after a few months in outpatient treatment. In addition to her individual psychotherapy, the patient also agreed to enter a group for women with eating disorders. She also has not had a migraine attack in 6 months.

Obesity—The technical definition of "obesity" is when body mass index (kg)/height (m^2) is above 30 or if body weight, by current standard charts, is at least 20% above the upper limit for height. In the medical–surgical inpatient setting, you will see situations of severe obesity, with weights ranging sometimes in the 300- to 500-lb (or more) range, which is referred to as *morbid obesity*.

Underlying endocrine and metabolic problems, brain tumors, and other disorders are ruled out initially as etiologic factors. Although it is established that there are strong genetic determinants to obesity, there also are important cultural and psychosocial influences.

Patients with obesity problems generally are treated by more than one discipline. It is very important to work with a nutritionist who can review the patient's diet and eating habits. It is useful to explore the psychosocial factors that are related to eating habits and ways for dealing with them. Frequently, this can be accomplished in special programs such as "Weight Watchers." Cognitive behavior therapy (CBT) is often particularly geared toward working with patients who have obesity problems. As is often the case with anorexia nervosa and bulimia nervosa, patients with severe obesity usually have a distorted body image and a distorted understanding of food, nutrition, weight, and topics dealing with being overweight or "fat." CBT treatment is ideally suited to help the patient restructure his or her thinking about these issues. Individual psychodynamic therapy may be helpful with some patients who are struggling with issues of dependency, self-esteem, and relationships. In our experience, these patients often use their extreme obesity to avoid sexual relationships. Specialized group therapy techniques are often an important part of the treatment plan. The newer antidepressants, particularly the selective serotonin reuptake inhibitors (SSRIs), have been shown to be helpful in binge eating disorders.

Typically, by the time you are called to see an obese patient in the hospital, there are usually significant medical sequelae. There may be plans to try special surgical techniques to bring about weight loss after other efforts have failed. One of the procedures used is a Roux-en-Y gastric bypass in which a line of staples is used to create a small pouch at the top of the stomach, which is then attached to the jejunum. This results in a bypass of most of the stomach and the duodenum. The patient must understand that this procedure radically reduces the amount of food that can be eaten at one time without getting very sick. There is also less area for nutrients to be absorbed. These patients risk developing a "dumping syndrome" where they become less tolerant of certain foods that enter the small intestine very quickly, and patients can develop nausea, faintness, and diarrhea, if the diet is not further altered.

Major surgical procedures usually are not recommended as cosmetic treatments, but they can be lifesaving to patients who have uncontrolled morbid obesity. Liposuction is a common cosmetic technique for abdominal obesity. As with other types of cosmetic surgery, inflated expectations for the procedure itself or how it can change the patients' lives can lead to depression and exacerbate underlying psychiatric disorders. Psychotherapy can be useful to patients with such issues, but the patient really has to be motivated for consultation and treatment.

We have found that the morbidly obese patient, when seen in the hospital, may present a management problem that can involve the staff as well as the patient.

CASE VIGNETTE: A VERY LARGE WEIGHT REQUIRES A VERY LARGE TEAM EFFORT

The patient is a 47-year-old man with diabetes mellitus and morbid obesity who was admitted for fainting spells. His weight was 450 lb approximately 2 years before his admission, but it was believed that he may have gained considerable weight since that time and the scales and logistics made it difficult to weigh the patient. He had a history of being married four times and having 10 children. His current girlfriend, who was also fairly obese, could not visit the patient because she was at their home, which was a 3-hour drive from the hospital. The patient had been a musician, but had not worked in several years. He had been treated for a bipolar condition several years previously with lithium, but had not followed up treatment. In the previous 2 years, he had rarely left the house and, in the last 6 months, he had not gotten out of bed. The patient did not show evidence of overt psychosis. He was provocative and seductive to female members of the staff and particularly to the medical students who were assigned to him. He would flirt, and the staff believed that he was exposing himself to them, although he denied such behavior. To complicate things more, he could barely walk or move around because of his obesity. He had to sleep and stay mostly on two mattresses that were moved together, as he took over a double room.

To better manage the situation, the patient was seen almost daily by the C-L psychiatrist. The C-L team held a series of meetings with the staff where various observations and complaints about the patient were aired. During some meetings, input was given by the staff as to the patient's reaction to the diet program that was being designed for him by the dietician, who allowed modifications to be made that were appreciated by the patient. The diabetologist was able to design a monitoring plan of the patient's glucose levels and insulin management that was suitable to the patient and ultimately stabilized some of the acute symptoms. There was a good deal of discussion and interaction among the staff at the meetings about the staff's reaction to the seductive and provocative behavior of the patient. Whereas some of the staff were very angry and dismissive of the patient and wanted him out of the hospital, others were sympathetic and saw him as very vulnerable, child-like, and frightened. There was a female medical student who initially had been spending a great deal of time talking to the patient, but then withdrew when he tried to be seductive. She was interested in trying to reengage the patient in a therapeutic manner. She set up supervisory sessions with one member of the C-L staff and resumed seeing the patient almost daily. She was very helpful in gaining the patient's cooperation for various procedures and getting him to accept some of the diet limitations. She handed the patient over to two other rotations of medical students (male and female) who worked closely with the patient under supervision. As the staff *began to appreciate the interest and concern that the C-L staff and some of the medical staff and nursing staff had for this patient, the overall approach to the patient clearly changed for the better. The patient's level of cooperation greatly improved. He was hospitalized for 3 to 4 months and lost considerable weight before he was transferred to a rehabilitation facility with a plan to return for gastric bypass surgery.*

LIAISON POTENTIAL

1. Work with the GI team or clinic and see their patients on a regular basis.
2. Become a part of the ID team and perform psychiatric evaluations of patients before start of hepatitis C therapy, provide follow-up and monitoring of patients on this regimen.
3. Become a consultant to patients with liver failure who are being considered for liver transplantation and patients and families before and after transplantation.
4. Work with an eating disorder multidisciplinary team in evaluating and treating patients with eating disorders.
5. Work with surgeons who do bariatric surgery, evaluating patients before and after surgery. Run groups for these types of patients.

Endocrinology and Autoimmune Disorders

9

Essential Concepts

- Just about all patients who are seen by a consulting psychiatrist should have their thyroid function tests (TFTs) reviewed.
- Previously treated hyperthyroidism, without continued replacement treatment, is an important cause of hypothyroidism.
- Calcium abnormalities suggest parathyroid gland dysfunction.
- Moon facies, truncal obesity, purple striae, buffalo hump, altered mood states, and sometimes psychosis are all stigmata of a hypercortisol state.
- Understanding the personal psychological meaning of diabetes mellitus to a patient may be just as important as figuring out the patient's insulin requirements.
- Patients with systemic lupus erythematosus (SLE) who have a delirium or other acute psychiatric symptoms while on steroids should have a differential diagnostic consideration between lupus cerebritis and steroid-induced mood disorder or steroid psychosis.

Most physicians do not think about calling a psychiatric consultant when they see patients who have conditions such as thyroid disease, diabetes mellitus, SLE, chronic fatigue syndrome (CFS), or other conditions that are mentioned in this chapter. However, these conditions, in fact, frequently have a significant psychiatric component. Patients who have these diseases often initially present with symptoms such as mood or behavior changes or even overt psychosis. It is your task as a consultation-liaison (C-L) psychiatrist to be able to include them in the differential diagnosis, when appropriate, and to know how to develop a treatment approach to their psychiatric manifestations.

THYROID DISEASE

Hypothyroidism

Every year, we diagnose a handful of previously undiagnosed cases of thyroid illness, both in our C-L inpatient work and in the course of doing outpatient consultations. Most of these cases are patients who have hypothyroidism who present with depression and/or cognitive deficits. They tend to be heavy set, often with gray hair, and can be in their 40s or older. One etiology, which is often not thought of, is previously treated hyperthyroidism. Such patients were treated by surgery or chemical ablation many years previously; they were given replacement hormones, which they subsequently stopped taking, leading eventually to hypothyroidism. Hashimoto's thyroid disease, which is probably secondary to an immune reaction, may be another common cause of hypothyroidism.

Most patients who present with depression and anxiety, who turn out to be hypothyroid, will respond very well to thyroxin replacement therapy. The lethargy, fatigue, and slowing of thought processes can be mistaken for a depressive disorder. If the hypothyroid state remains untreated, the patient can become overtly psychotic and this state, in past years, was called *myxedema madness*. In addition to blood tests, it is useful to have a sonogram to rule out underlying cancer. Radioactive isotope tests can be done to demonstrate the proper functioning of the thyroid and to diagnose cold spots, which would be suspicious of cancer. Patients treated with replacement thyroxin may have complete resolution of their depression or it may persist and require the use of antidepressants, with or without psychotherapy.

Hyperthyroidism and Graves' Disease

Hyperthyroidism can present with anxiety, sweating, tremor, racing thoughts, and hyperactivity. Such patients also may present with labile affect and become paranoid, manic, or have other psychotic manifestations. While the most common cause of hyperthyroidism is Graves' disease, it also can occur in situations where large doses of thyroid hormone are being administered without proper monitoring.

The bottom line here is that just about all patients who are being seen by a consulting psychiatrist should have TFTs. The best indicator of thyroid dysfunction is usually thyroid-stimulating hormone (TSH), with low levels indicating hyperthyroidism and high levels indicating hypothyroidism. Never be reluctant to request or even insist on TFTs, even if you are 90% sure that the patient has a treatable psychiatric condition. Never assume that the patient's outside doctor must have checked out this possibility.

CASE VIGNETTE: THYROID DISEASE PRESENTS AS HIGH ANXIETY

The C-L consultant was called to the medical emergency room (ER) to see a 35-year-old man who was hyperventilating and believed to have anxiety and panic symptoms. The patient was currently in a cognitive behavior program for panic disorder. He also would occasionally use diazepam (Valium) (5 mg) to relieve his anxiety. He described being anxious most of the time, with occasional episodes of sweating a great deal and feeling his heart beat fast. He would become scared and breathe rapidly during these episodes. He also was afraid that something terrible was happening to him and there was a suggestion of paranoia, although his reality testing was good. Physical examination was normal, except for slightly elevated blood pressure and tachycardia of 120, which also showed on electrocardiogram (ECG) with sinus rhythm. The C-L consultant noted that the patient had a fine tremor of both hands. The patient felt much better after receiving 1 mg of alprazolam (Xanax) and rebreathing into a bag. He was referred to both medical and psychiatry clinics for follow-up. On a hunch of the consultant, TFTs were drawn before he left the ER. The tests later confirmed hyperthyroidism. The patient eventually was referred for endocrine consultation and diagnosed with Graves' disease. He was treated and showed marked improvement in anxiety and stress symptoms. He did not require further treatment for panic symptoms.

Lithium and Thyroid Disease

Lithium, which is commonly used to treat bipolar disorder, can interfere with thyroid metabolism and can cause hypothyroidism. Therefore, when seeing such patients, include TFTs in their monitoring laboratory tests and observe for the development of a goiter.

PARATHYROID DISEASE

Although much less common than thyroid disease, parathyroid disease can present with psychiatric symptoms, such as depression, irritability, anxiety, confusion, and delirium.

Hyperparathyroidism

Elevated calcium is the tip-off that the patient might have hyperparathyroidism. Excessive parathyroid hormone causes abnormal regulation of calcium metabolism and subsequent hypercalcemia. Muscle weakness also can be part of the presentation.

Hypoparathyroidism

Low calcium levels go along with hypoparathyroid disorders, which can cause similar symptoms, as mentioned earlier. Tetany may be present with low calcium, but might not be present if the calcium is gradually lowered. Seizures can occur, as can cataract formation.

It is possible to get an assay of parathyroid hormone, which can be helpful in the diagnosis of parathyroid disease. Both magnesium and phosphate levels can be abnormal, but calcium is usually the key test. Psychiatric symptoms can be expected to improve as the parathyroid condition is treated.

ADRENAL GLAND DYSFUNCTION

Cortisol-releasing factor (CRF) from the hypothalamus causes the release of adrenocorticotropic hormone (ACTH) from the anterior pituitary gland and then cortisol from the adrenal gland. Excessive CRF may produce Cushing's disease, whereas

CRF deficiency may cause diminished cortisol production and Addison's disease.

Hypercortisol State—Cushing's Disease/Syndrome

Cushing's syndrome is the term used for any clinical pattern that is secondary to elevated cortisol whether it is endogenous or exogenous. The clinical picture usually is recognized easily. The patient has moon facies, truncal obesity (in fact, the obesity is often part of the reason for the consultation, if the patient is an outpatient), and may have purple striae and a buffalo hump. The patient also can have osteoporosis, proximal muscle weakness, and hirsutism. There can be a full range of mood changes from manic lability to depression. Suicidality is a possibility and the patient can be psychotic. The patient with Cushing's syndrome also can have a delirium, and this condition always should be part of the differential diagnosis of delirium.

Although depression is more likely with Cushing's disease, hypomanic or manic symptoms are more likely with exogenous steroids. In its most severe form, this syndrome is known as *steroid psychosis*. Mood changes can occur at any dosage of steroids, but significant mood changes are more likely to occur at higher doses (i.e., more than 30 mg of prednisone).

CASE VIGNETTE: MENTAL STATUS IN BODYBUILDERS WHO USE STEROIDS

A psychiatric consultation was requested for a 28-year-old man who was just admitted after sustaining a compound fracture of the tibia in a motor vehicle accident, which needed to be set in the operating room (OR). Shortly after recovering from anesthesia and being transferred to the orthopedic unit, he was noted to be saying strange things. He had rapid speech and was grandiose, announcing that he was the "third strongest man in the world." He knew where he was and the date, but he had rapid and somewhat pressured speech and obviously was not concentrating very well. He denied any psychiatric history and gave a history of being a motorcycle mechanic. Drug and alcohol levels were normal on admission. The preliminary diagnosis was delirium secondary to pain medication. Head injury also was considered, although brain imaging was normal

*on admission and the patient had not lost consciousness. The
patient gave permission to contact his family who had just
left the hospital. They confirmed that the patient had never
had psychiatric treatment and, as far as they knew, he did
not drink excessively or take drugs. They reported that for
the previous 2 weeks he had appeared distracted and had not
been his usual self. They thought that he was not sleeping well.
They said that he spent all of his spare time working out at
the gymnasium and that he had been in some bodybuilding
contests. In retrospect, the consultant realized that the patient
was quite muscular. The patient was then questioned about
his bodybuilding efforts. He described using many vitamins
and special supplements. He said that all of his friends used
anabolic steroids and he acknowledged that he did, as well.
For the past month, he had started using a new version of a
steroid that everyone said was the best. It was then clear that
the patient had steroid-induced psychosis and mood disorder.*

Hypocortisol State—Addison's Disease

This condition usually is due to chronic adrenocortical atrophy, but it can be caused by a granulomatous disease, such as tuberculosis. Diminished cortisol will produce apathy and easy fatigability, which may be difficult to distinguish from depression. The treatment is administration of exogenous corticosteroids.

DIABETES MELLITUS

In our experience, patients with diabetes mellitus present with psychological issues that are related to the following three different phases of the illness:

1. Onset
2. Adjustment
3. Crisis

Onset of Diabetes Mellitus

Informing a person that he or she has a chronic serious illness is a major life event. Typical psychological reactions include denial, anxiety, and depression. Therefore, you need to be alert to the fact that a symptomatic patient may be reacting to the impact of a recent diagnosis. Because diabetes can have genetic links, it is important to understand what the experience and course of the illness of other family members may have been. When regular injections of insulin are required, patients who are phobic of needles may require some desensitization techniques to help them accept this process. Some patients will find the dietary restrictions very difficult to follow because of eating patterns and carbohydrate craving, which can be closely linked to the patient's psychological makeup. The patient also may require psychoeducation, behavior modification, and psychological exploration. Adolescents may find it particularly disruptive to change diet patterns, which can give them a sense of being "different" and not fitting in with their peers.

The use of oral hypoglycemic agents, state-of-the-art equipment for home testing of blood sugar levels, and a more sophisticated approach to the use of insulin has mitigated some of the initial psychological problems that are seen after the onset of this illness. Nonetheless, the ideal approach for a newly diagnosed diabetic patient takes into account the personality style of the patient and matches it with the management of insulin. For example, a very rigid obsessive compulsive person might be treated best with a very strict diet and insulin schedule, whereas a patient with a more flexible personality style might be comfortable with a more flexible management approach.

Adjustment to Diabetes Mellitus

Some of the issues described in the preceding text might not become apparent until the patient has lived with the disease and treatment for a while. It is almost inevitable that some patients, particularly adolescents with diabetes, will wonder eventually if they can function without insulin. Such patients, at some point, go off their diet or stop using insulin or both to see if they "really need" this treatment. Eventually there is usually a dangerous hyperglycemic problem, which often occurs immediately after the initial experimentation.

Although people with diabetes often have increased levels of anxiety and depression, there is still some controversy as to whether increased stress leads to increased glucose levels. Whether or not altered psychological states directly lead to changes in glucose metabolism, it is certainly possible that psychological states that lead to distraction can lead to failure to properly test the blood or administer insulin with subsequent physical consequences. Patients with borderline personality disorder may choose to manipulate others by improper control of their own insulin.

Crisis

Patients in diabetic ketoacidosis or insulin shock often are unconscious when they are seen initially by a physician. The differential diagnosis is grounded in basic emergency medicine, and you will rarely be called upon to make such clinical decisions in your capacity as a psychiatrist. However, in some clinical situations, diabetic ketoacidosis can be confused with psychiatric disorders, such as catatonia, conversion symptoms, mutism, malingering, or anxious hyperventilation. In addition, both hypoglycemia and hyperglycemia can present as classical delirium. When in doubt, a simple blood test will make the diagnosis.

Injection of insulin can be used as a suicide attempt or even as attempted murder. You will need to rely on history and clinical acumen to sniff out these unusual circumstances and then act accordingly.

It has been shown that there is a high association between depression and diabetes. Depression has a significant impact on the quality of life and compliance with the management of diabetes. There also appears to be depression-induced changes in the hypothalamic-pituitary axis that result in metabolic changes that would ultimately affect glucose control. This is why you should be vigilant in recognizing the depression, which is often underrecognized in this cohort of patients. In the collaborative model of depression management in primary care, attention has been given to the mental health of patients with HgbA1C greater than 9 despite treatment. There are several medical complications of diabetes mellitus, including heart disease, stroke, and renal disease; the potential psychological ramifications of these are discussed elsewhere in this book. One particularly dramatic complication of severe diabetes is amputation, which is caused by peripheral vascular disease. Sometimes there is progressive gangrene, which requires a series of amputations of digits, toes, and eventually limbs. Similarly, there can be a progressive loss of vision over time due to diabetic retinopathy. No matter how well adjusted or prepared a patient may seem to be for such complications, you must appreciate that the patient has undergone a major loss of self and function. Along with the grief, there is demoralization and depression. The patient should be allowed to grieve and go through the phases of bereavement. As with any grieving process, the therapeutic skills of listening, clarification, and empathy will be much more valuable than a simple prescription of a tranquilizer or an antidepressant. However, adjunctive medication always can be considered and, at times, is quite helpful.

CASE VIGNETTE: DIABETES CAN HIT HARD, ESPECIALLY TO A TEENAGER

A C-L consultation was called for a 17-year-old teenager who was thought to be having a rough time in managing her diabetes. She was described by her doctor as "a good kid, very bright, who had learned all about diabetes but was having unstable fluctuations of her glucose that were difficult to control." She had been admitted to the hospital in insulin shock, after what was believed to be an accidental overdose of insulin. The referring doctor thought that the patient might be a candidate for a newly forming group for adolescents with chronic illness and suggested that the consultant "come by and talk to her about the group." The patient was an attractive sullen teenager who initially had nothing much to say. The consultant engaged the patient on a variety of subjects that were unrelated to her diabetes, which included movies, music, school, analysis of colleges, and various careers. By the time the consultant got around to asking her about how she handled her diagnosis of diabetes, the patient was quite comfortable with the consultant. She related that she was devastated by the diet, revolted by the needles, and scared that she was going to go blind from diabetes, as had her grandmother. She felt that her parents did not know what they were talking about when they reassured her. She tried to hide the fact of her illness from her friends and was afraid to go to the beach because her needle marks might show. She also could not imagine being intimate with her boyfriend for the same reason. She experimented with not using insulin and by eating hardly anything, and, at other times, she would eat "all the wrong foods." She was becoming increasingly depressed and had not slept well for the previous 2 weeks. She had fantasies of injecting too much insulin and being rescued by a handsome doctor in the ER. At other times, she thought of injecting too much insulin and "going to sleep forever." She thought maybe she purposely injected too much insulin the night that she was brought to the hospital. The patient began to sob and said that she felt relieved that she had shared her feelings. She asked if the consultant would help her tell her parents how she felt, and she agreed to see a therapist and attend the group for young diabetics that the consultant was coleading.

SYSTEMIC LUPUS ERYTHEMATOSUS

SLE is a multisystem autoimmune disease that can have significant psychiatric implications. Although the intricacies of the illness are still being elucidated, SLE can produce a vasculitis in just about every part of the body, leading to symptoms, such as fever, photosensitivity, butterfly rash, joint pain, and headaches. More serious but common symptoms include anemia, pleural effusion, renal failure, seizures, and many psychiatric symptoms that are related to the impact on the central nervous system. The latter symptoms usually are attributed to "lupus cerebritis," which, in the full-blown presentation, would be seen as a classic delirium with disturbance of consciousness, reduced ability to maintain attention, memory problems, disorientation, and even hallucinations (visual more likely than auditory). The patient also can present with depressive symptoms, including insomnia, irritability, emotional lability, and suicidal ideation.

The term *lupus* derives from the root meaning "wolf" and the presentation and manifestations of this condition can be as "sly and cunning" as its namesake. For example, the delirium may not be due to lupus cerebritis, but it may be due to renal failure and uremia. The depression may not be due to the direct effect of the medical condition, but could be a psychological reaction to this illness, which most often strikes at young women who are on the threshold of their mature lives and takes away their health.

To further complicate the clinical picture, steroids are used to treat acute episodes of SLE and can themselves cause significant changes in mood, as well as psychotic manifestations or a delirium. Sometimes you may actually be the first person to suggest that an antinuclear antibody ANA test or other tests to diagnose SLE be done. But, even if you arrive on the scene when the patient is already known to have SLE, there may be a dilemma as to whether the psychiatric manifestations are due to SLE cerebritis or steroid treatment. A very close look at the timeline of the symptoms and treatment may give some clues. A basic test, such as serial erythrocyte sedimentation rate ESR, may indicate whether the SLE disease process is improving or worsening and, therefore, may help with the differential diagnosis.

CASE VIGNETTE: LUPUS PSYCHOSIS VERSUS STEROID PSYCHOSIS

A psychiatric consultation was called on a 33-year-old woman with a known diagnosis of SLE who was noted to be crying in bed and threatening to kill herself. She also was acting paranoid and was fearful of the patient in the next bed. The medical and nursing staff were very upset by the degree of her psychological stress. She had been admitted to the hospital 10 days before consultation, with pleural effusion and multiple joint pains. She was felt to have an exacerbation of her SLE and, on admission, she was put on prednisone and the dosage was titrated up to 80 mg per day. The treating physicians thought that the patient was having a steroid psychosis. In view of the patient's improving joint symptoms and pleural effusion, they told the psychiatrist that they were willing to reduce the steroids to relieve the psychiatric symptoms. The psychiatrist found that the patient was having psychotic manifestations that included paranoid delusions about her family and auditory hallucinations—voices telling her that she was evil. She was disoriented to time and place and could not do simple calculations. The family who was visiting at the bedside gave a history that the patient had been functioning very well for many years, working as an advertising executive, and on no medications. Two weeks before admission, she began to act strange, was irritable and forgetful, and began to accuse her family of talking about her behind her back. Her physical symptoms then developed and she was admitted to the hospital. The electroencephalogram (EEG) that was taken on the day of the C-L consultation was checked by the C-L consultant, with the neurologist, and found to be abnormal, with marked diffuse slowing. Renal function was normal. The C-L consultant concluded that the most probable cause of the patient's psychiatric symptoms was lupus cerebritis. She spoke with the treating team and told them that, most probably, the steroids were not the main cause of the patient's psychiatric symptoms and, in fact, that they were probably going to be helpful in relieving the symptoms. She suggested the addition of a combination of haloperidol and risperidone to treat the patient's delirium and psychotic manifestations. She also attempted to do some reality testing and supportive care with the patient. She met regularly with the family until the patient was able to go into remission of her SLE. It also was recommended, at that time, that the steroids be tapered gradually to avoid further psychiatric symptoms that can occur with a rapid steroid withdrawal.

CHRONIC FATIGUE SYNDROME

Fatigue is one of the most common of patient complaints. Oftentimes, when the etiology of the fatigue is unexplainable, a diagnosis of CFS is given. Unfortunately, this does not clear up the situation, as there are controversies surrounding this diagnosis. There is no clear consensus regarding diagnostic criteria or etiology of CFS. In its earlier days, CFS was linked to finding antibodies of Epstein-Barr virus (EBV), but this was later found to be a weak link.

As a C-L psychiatrist, you will be called to see patients with chronic fatigue where workup has not revealed any significant etiology. Many different medical and psychiatric conditions that are associated with fatigue need to be excluded. Depression is always in the differential diagnosis. There is a tendency to order an extensive workup and you need to be cautious in recommending tests. Although the patient starts off in the hospital, by the time CFS is under serious consideration, the patient has been converted to an outpatient.

Unfortunately, most patients with CFS are not receptive to psychiatric intervention, despite studies that show a high comorbidity with psychiatric conditions. This has been perpetuated by the popular media and some practitioners who have fostered the belief that there is a purely physical reason for this fatigue.

What you need to do as a C-L psychiatrist is to get an accurate history, establish a supportive relationship with the patient, validate the patient's suffering, and treat the underlying psychiatric conditions where they exist. Often, the patient is not receptive to considering that the fatigue may have a psychological origin. They are much more likely to be interested in talking about the discouragement and depression that they feel from being limited or incapacitated by their symptoms. If the patient engages in a psychotherapeutic relationship even around these issues, there then may be the opportunity to find underlying psychological factors. At the very least, giving the patient empathic support may be quite helpful.

FIBROMYALGIA

Fibromyalgia is another one of the nonspecific conditions that presents with chronic fatigue and should be included in the differential. The Centers for Disease Control and Prevention (CDC) has suggested that fibromyalgia is a subset of CFS. Unlike CFS, however, studies have shown that antidepressants can improve fibromyalgia.

LIAISON POTENTIAL

1. Be a psychiatric consultant to an endocrine team. Make rounds with them and see all patients who have thyroid disease or other conditions that are followed by the team.
2. Work closely with diabetologists and members of the team that follow up patients who have diabetes mellitus. See the patients during each phase of the illness and assist with adjustment to the condition.
3. Work closely with a rheumatologist or a group and see all or most of their patients who have SLE and other autoimmune disorders, especially during acute phases.
4. If there is a team of specialists who are trying to work with patients who have CFS, they may be quite receptive to having a C-L psychiatrist work with them.

**Psychiatric Aspects
of Neurologic Disorders**

Essential Concepts

- The hallmark of delirium is the inability to attend and not the fluctuation of mental status or disorientation.
- Not all dementias present the same way and some present as if there were no cognitive impairment at all. Early in the course of subcortical dementias, the patient may score 30/30 on the Folstein Mini-Mental Status Examination and yet, on neuropsychological testing, may show significant cognitive deficits.
- Dementia is the effect of pathologic processes in the brain, not the effect of aging.
- When using psychotropics in patients who have had insults to the brain from whatever etiology, always *"start low and go slow."*

The presence of pathological lesions in the brain can be expected to cause psychiatric manifestations. In the past, these lesions were grouped under the terms *organic brain disorders* or *organic mental syndromes.* Often they were compared with the "functional disorders" that were believed not to have an underlying organic etiology. We now know that the so-called functional mental disorders, such as schizophrenia and bipolar disorder, actually have an organic basis. Organic mental disorders, so named because there is an organic basis in the form of a medical or surgical disorder or some other pathology, include delirium, dementia, amnesic disorders, and various psychiatric disorders that are primarily caused by a general medical condition. Diagnostic and Statistical Manual of Mental Disorders, Fourth Edition (DSM-IV) classifies this group of disorders as "cognitive disorders" to emphasize the common element in all of them: the presence of cognitive impairment.

Parkinson's disease (PD), multiple sclerosis (MS), and cerebrovascular accidents (CVAs) are some neurologic disorders that are often so intertwined with psychiatric symptoms and vice versa. In the chapter on cancer, we referred to primary and metastatic lesions in the brain. It is important to know how to correlate the psychiatric and neurologic manifestations and to distinguish whether the patient's symptoms are of neurologic or psychiatric origin.

DELIRIUM

Delirium is one of the most common psychiatric disorders in a general hospital. It is also often misdiagnosed and underrecognized. The prevalence has been shown to vary from 10% to 50% in medical–surgical units. It is important to recognize this entity as soon as possible because it is often a medical emergency. Perhaps conceptualizing delirium as an "acute brain failure" will convey the sense of urgency that is necessary when evaluating these cases. There are certain cases of delirium that need to be recognized immediately because they can lead to death (Table 10.1).

There are several patient groups who are at increased risk to develop delirium: patients who are very young or very old, with third-degree burns, with a substance dependence history, who are status post cardiotomy, who have a history of preexisting brain damage, or who have a history of delirium. One of the first things you should do when you get a consult request to evaluate a patient who has mental status changes is to review the chart. It is important to look through the patient's laboratory results, medications (paying attention to the medication changes and the anticholinergic load of medications

TABLE 10.1. WHHHHIMP Mnemonic of Some Serious Etiologies of Delirium

---

□ Withdrawal from drugs/alcohol/Wernicke's encephalopathy
□ Hypertensive encephalopathy
□ Hypoglycemia
□ Hypoperfusion of central nervous system
□ Hypoxemia
□ Intracranial bleeding
□ Meningitis/encephalitis
□ Poisons/medications

---

that the patient is on), nurses' notes, and the patient's vital signs. Arterial blood gases (ABGs) and blood glucose results are essential for evaluating a patient to determine the etiology of the delirium. If these tests have not yet been ordered and hypoglycemia and hypoxemia are high in the differential list, you should recommend that they be done. Renal, liver, and thyroid function tests also should be taken into account.

Clinical Features of Delirium

Delirium is a clinical syndrome and, as such, presents with varied clinical features. These features may not all be present in a single patient. However, there is a core symptom of delirium that should be present before it can be diagnosed and this is the inability to attend, which is the inability to shift, focus, or sustain attention.

CASE VIGNETTE: AN ANGRY HOSTILE MAN WHO NEEDED OXYGEN

A 72-year-old man was "wreaking havoc" in the unit. He was demanding to be discharged against medical advice. He was a pleasant man who had chronic obstructive pulmonary disease (COPD) and hypertension (HTN). He was admitted for weakness and fatigue and was being worked up. He had been in the hospital for 3 days, when he went to the nursing station in his wheelchair and insisted on being discharged at once. A psychiatric consult was requested. When the psychiatrist evaluated him, the patient was quite hostile and was incensed that people thought he was "crazy" because the staff had called a psychiatrist. He did oblige and answered the questions. He was awake and oriented to time, place, and person. He was not overtly delusional or hallucinating. His memory was intact, but he was noted to be quite distractible and did not focus on the psychiatrist and his questions. He wanted to be discharged because there was "nothing wrong with him." ABGs taken just before his outburst revealed hypoxemia. The patient was given oxygen and, approximately an hour later, he was much calmer and agreed to stay.

The course of delirium is acute and there may be a prodrome. A review of the nurses' notes may reveal a reversal of the patient's sleep patterns and this precedes the confusion that often leads to a psychiatric consultation request. Fluctuation of mental status, although not necessarily found in all cases, is a common feature of delirium. By the time you get called, the patient may already be lucid. You should review the records to have a longitudinal history that will give you the whole picture.

A patient does not need to be totally disoriented to be diagnosed with delirium, as long as there is the inability to attend, which is the core symptom of delirium. However, most patients with delirium are disoriented and also present with other neurologic symptoms (e.g., abnormal reflexes). Other features of delirium include perceptual disturbances, such as delusions, hallucinations, and illusions. Some hallucinations indicate certain diagnostic entities (e.g., olfactory hallucinations may suggest a brain tumor, kinesthetic hallucinations suggest drug withdrawal, etc.). There can be mood disturbances, disorganized thoughts, and deficits in language and cognition (memory, concentration, etc.). Delirium can be hyperactive, where the patient is quite agitated and poses a behavior management problem. This type of delirious patient often is the reason for stat psychiatric consults.

The other type is hypoactive delirium and, unfortunately, it is often missed. The patient is often just lying in bed, appearing depressed and apathetic. If a psychiatric consult is called, it is usually for depression. This is often the reason why delirium is misdiagnosed. Hypoactive delirium is the more dangerous type because the etiology for the delirium is not recognized, and therefore not treated.

There are several available rating scales for delirium (the revised version of the Trepacz Delirium Rating Scale, the Memorial Delirium Assessment Scale, among others). The Folstein Mini-Mental Status Examination is a screening tool that is often used, but it is not specific for delirium. Simple bedside tests also can help reach a diagnosis, such as alternate hand movements and draw-a-clock tests. The diagnosis is best arrived at by doing a good clinical examination.

Management of Delirium

The most important aspect of managing the delirious patient is finding the etiology and correcting or treating the problem. Oftentimes, the etiology is multifactorial. In hyperactive delirium, the patient may not be cooperative and could be too agitated to allow for a workup to establish the etiology of delirium. In these situations, you need to start symptomatic management of the delirium. There is still some controversy regarding the administration of neuroleptics in delirium as to whether they should be given as a standing order, as needed, or not at all. A more recent school of thought advocates the use of neuroleptics in hypoactive delirium. This relates more to the treatment of the cognitive impairments that are seen in all types of delirium. Low-dose haloperidol has been the first-line drug that is used. For example, start at 0.5 mg twice a day (b.i.d.) by mouth (PO) and titrate upward and, eventually, discontinue the drug when there is no need for it. The fact that it can be given through various routes [(oral, intramuscularly (IM), and intravenously (IV)] makes it more widely used. It is important to remember that haloperidol is not approved by the U.S. Food and Drug Administration (FDA) for IV administration, nor is it labeled as indicated for delirium. An uncommon, but significant, complication of IV haloperidol is *torsades de pointes* (cardiac arrhythmia with QT prolongation). More recently, there have been anecdotal reports and a few studies that show that low doses of risperidone, olanzapine, and even quetiapine can be used to treat delirium. Aside from the neuroleptics, benzodiazepines, particularly lorazepam, also are used for the agitation that is seen in delirium. Often, lorazepam is used in combination with neuroleptics, and, in other cases, it is used alone. Lorazepam should be the drug of choice in cases of delirium that are caused by drug or alcohol withdrawal. In addition to pharmacologic management, environmental manipulation, such as repeatedly orienting the patient, having familiar objects around, having a nightlight, having someone around and so forth, also are part of the management of the delirious patient. Never lose sight of the fact that attention must be directed toward finding the underlying etiology and treating it.

DEMENTIA

Dementia is a syndrome of acquired and persistent impairment in intellectual functioning that affects memory, language, visuospatial skills, emotion or personality, and cognition. It is important to remember that dementia is the effect of pathological processes in the brain, not the effect of aging. As the population in the United States ages, however, the prevalence of dementia will increase. The diagnosis of dementia is based on the patient's history and clinical presentation.

Clinical Features of Dementia

The clinical presentation of dementia can be conceptualized into three domains: cognitive, functional, and behavioral. Cognitive symptoms include memory impairment, the four As (amnesia, aphasia, apraxia, and agnosia), impaired executive functioning, and visuospatial dysfunction, among others. Behavioral symptoms include sadness, irritability, and anxiety early in the course of the disease. Agitation, wandering behavior, delusions and hallucinations, and sleeplessness occur later in the course of the disease. In the early stages, functional activities that are affected include cooking, housekeeping, traveling independently, handling finances, and so forth. These are also called *instrumental activities of daily living* (IADLs). Personal activities of daily living (ADLs) (e.g., bathing, toileting, dressing, and eating, etc.) are affected later.

Dementia can be cortical, subcortical, and mixed. Cortical dementia is best typified by Alzheimer's disease (AD), in which memory impairment is the most significant cognitive deficit. Approximately 90% of patients with dementia have a lifetime risk of significant psychopathology. Flattened sulci, enlarged ventricles, and diffuse atrophy are noted on imaging studies. Autopsy shows neurofibrillary tangles and amyloid plaques. The course is a gradually progressive deterioration in cognition, function, and behavior.

In subcortical dementia, apathy, depression, and psychomotor retardation are more prominent than is memory impairment. The frontal lobe, basal ganglia, and thalamus are affected. The dementias of various illnesses, such as human immunodeficiency virus (HIV) and PD are subcortical dementias.

Multi-infarct dementia (MID) or vascular dementia (VD) are mixed types of dementia. This means that they have features of both cortical and subcortical types. In VD, there is a stepwise deterioration of functioning that correlates with each vascular event. There also can be some degree of improvement after each event. Imaging studies often show multiple parenchymal lesions scattered all over. A combination of AD and VD is not uncommon.

There are two other types of dementia that have been increasingly recognized of late Lewy body dementia and frontotemporal dementia. Lewy body dementia is often combined with AD or VD. The core feature is the fluctuating cognition that looks much like a delirium, persistent visual hallucinations, and parkinsonism. Frontotemporal dementia or Pick's disease is characterized by atrophy of the frontal and temporal lobes and results in a distinct pattern of poor social skills, disinhibition, impulsivity, apathy and aphasias, and hyperorality.

Personality changes and perceptual disturbances are part of the picture of the different dementias. The phenomenon of "sundowning," increased confusion toward the end of the day, is another common clinical feature of the dementias.

Pseudodementia is the dementia syndrome of depression and deserves mention here, as it should be considered in the differential diagnosis. Patients who have pseudodementia are indifferent to their symptoms of cognitive impairment, unlike cortically demented individuals who are distressed by the fact that they have impaired cognition. The patient often gives "I don't know" answers. Attention and concentration are well preserved in pseudodementia. This "dementia" improves when depression is treated.

Management of Dementia

There is really no cure for most dementias, but they certainly are treatable. The drugs currently available for the management of dementia actually do not cure the dementia, but they do retard the progressive deterioration of the patient's cognitive status and, in some cases, also improve the patient's behavioral symptoms and, as a result, improve the patient's functioning. The drugs include the cholinesterase inhibitors donepezil, rivastigmine, and galantamine. Tacrine was the first of this type of drug, but it had a host of side effects that have precluded its use. Memantine, an N-methyl-D-aspartate (NMDA) receptor antagonist, is the first of a different class of drugs now used to treat the symptoms of AD. It is often used in combination with the cholinesterase inhibitors, most commonly donepezil. There are other drugs (e.g., selegiline, hydergine, etc.) antioxidant vitamins (vitamin E) and minerals, and complementary medicines (e.g., ginkgo biloba) that have been used, but, at present, there is no evidence-based literature to back up their efficacy. Low-dose antipsychotics, mood stabilizers, antidepressants, and antianxiety agents have been used to target specific symptoms that accompany a patient's dementia. It is essential to remember that patients with dementia can be particularly sensitive to side effects of medications and are usually on a number of medications that could interact with the psychotropics. In addition, it is important to identify the specific target symptom that you would want to treat with a particular psychotropic medication. Up to approximately 60% of patients with AD have depressive symptoms and, most often, they are underrecognized. Treatment of the depression can sometimes lead to an improvement in mood and functioning. Nonpharmacologic approaches to the management of AD are the cornerstone of treatment. This includes psychoeducation targeted at patients and their families, aids to help patients with their memory, and individual or group therapy, among others.

AMNESIC DISORDERS

In contrast to delirium and dementia where there are several cognitive impairments in the presenting symptoms, amnesic disorders only have one cognitive impairment: memory. Both retrograde (the inability to retain information learned) and anterograde (the inability to learn new information) memory can be impaired. The key is that this memory impairment significantly affects the patient's functioning. The causes of amnesic disorder are usually systemic medical illnesses, primary brain disorders, and substance-related causes (e.g., alcohol or benzodiazepines). The treatment of amnesic disorders primarily involves finding out the etiology and addressing the management of the cause. Psychotherapy also is helpful sometimes, as the patient feels overwhelmed by an awareness of memory deficits.

PARKINSON'S DISEASE

PD is a very common degenerative disorder, the prevalence of which increases with increasing age. Its pathogenesis is related to acetylcholine and dopamine depletion. It is a progressive disorder with a high prevalence of psychiatric manifestations. The features of PD are bradykinesia, rigidity, tremor at rest, gait abnormality, and dysfunction of posture and balance.

The most common psychiatric feature of PD is depression which has been reported to be as high as 40%. There have been studies that suggest that patients with PD are more depressed than similarly disabled patients with other medical illnesses. Depression can be the presenting symptom of PD. There is no solid data that shows a relationship between severity of the motor illness and the severity of depression. In the treatment of depression in patients with PD, selective serotonin reuptake inhibitors (SSRIs) are usually first-line drugs. You need to be aware, however, of the possible interaction between selegiline, an antiparkinsonian drug that is a selective monoamine oxidase (MAOI) B inhibitor, and SSRIs. Like other severely depressed medically ill patients, electroconvulsive therapy (ECT) can be a good treatment option if medications are not effective.

Anxiety is another common psychiatric symptom in patients with PD. In most cases, it is comorbid with depression. It can be quite disabling and more than just a reaction to the illness. Treatment is similar to that for others who have anxiety without PD.

PD also is associated with cognitive deficits, which suggest a subcortical dementia that presents with impairment in executive functioning. Using cholinesterase inhibitors in PD dementia may lead to a worsening of the patient's symptoms, thereby causing a decline in functioning. Lewy body dementia, a variant of PD, is more of a cortical dementia that is similar to AD.

Recently, it was noted that sleep disturbances are also manifestations of PD. These include insomnia, excessive daytime sleepiness, and sleep attacks, These can further impair patients and are associated with nighttime hallucinations and agitation.

Anticholinergic and dopaminergic agents that are used to treat PD may lead to delusions, hallucinations, mania, anxiety, and confusion. Delusions are persecutory in nature. Visual hallucinations are a common side effect of medications that are used to treat PD. Confusion particularly occurs in patients with preexisting cognitive impairment who are on anticholinergic drugs.

CEREBROVASCULAR ACCIDENTS

CVAs, or strokes, are among the most common causes of mortality and morbidity in the elderly in the United States. Most strokes are due to cerebral infarctions that are caused by thromboembolic phenomena. A smaller percentage of strokes are due to intracerebral hemorrhage and/or subarachnoid hemorrhage.

Most patients with a stroke exhibit contralateral weakness or paralysis of the upper and lower extremities, whereas a few have sensory deficits. The neurologic features of strokes usually are related to the location of the lesion. Among the most common psychiatric features of CVAs are pathologic emotional expressions of depression, mania, and anxiety. By this, we mean expression of emotions that are not directly linked to a mood that the patient is feeling. Pathologic emotions in a stroke victim are different from pseudobulbar palsy in that there is no paralysis of the voluntary muscles of the face. Pathologic crying or laughing is not provoked by any stimuli. When it occurs, there is no relationship to any mood change before, during, or after the expression of pathologic crying or laughing. A few studies have shown that antidepressants (e.g., nortriptyline, citalopram, fluoxetine, and sertraline) are effective in reducing poststroke pathologic crying.

It is a well-known fact that there is a link between the occurrence of a stroke and the subsequent development of depression. The prevalence of depression following an acute CVA ranges from 20% to 50%. The controversy lies in whether the location of the lesion has a relationship with the occurrence of depression. That is, those patients with lesions in the left frontal region and the left basal ganglia are more likely to develop a major depression. There is also the thought that persons who are depressed have a higher risk of developing a stroke. Several studies have shown that antidepressants work for patients with poststroke depression. ECT has been reported to be effective for poststroke depression. Psychostimulants also have been used with good effect. Nonpharmacologic management of depression, such as group, individual, and cognitive behavioral therapy, is helpful and should be tried. Whether or not the mood and its expression have been brought about by the location of the damaged brain, you should be able to recognize that the patient with a CVA usually has suffered severe losses in many spheres. These losses include motor and cognitive deficits that may impair the ability of the person to function as a parent, grandparent, or a useful member of society. This can be quite devastating and can account for the degree of depression that the patient may suffer.

MULTIPLE SCLEROSIS

MS is an autoimmune disease that is one of the most common causes of disability involving the nervous system in young adults. The neurologic features often involve many different sensory and motor functions. It is a chronic disease that has several patterns: the relapsing–remitting form, where acute attacks occur and disability accumulates over time; the secondary progressive form, where the initial phase is relapsing and remitting, followed by progression of the disease with increasing disability; the primary progressive form, where the disease is progressive from the outset; and the progressive relapsing form, where the disease starts as progressive with overlapping relapses.

MS is more common in women, and the age of onset is younger for women (late 20s). Diagnosis depends on the history and the clinical examination, which includes an extensive neurologic examination. Magnetic resonance imaging (MRI) can be important in confirming the diagnosis, as well as in monitoring the course of the disease. Neurologic features include visual problems that could lead to blindness; gait and balance problems that could progress to paraparesis, spasticity, and ataxia; sensory syndromes; bowel and bladder dysfunction; and cognitive deficits, particularly recent memory, sustained attention, speed of cognitive processing, and conceptual reasoning. At times, this condition can present with transient visual symptoms and no other signs or symptoms for many years. There is a high prevalence of depression in this population (14% to 57% in different studies), particularly in those who have the relapsing–remitting course. MS is a progressive and unpredictable illness. However, the degree of physical disability because of the illness does not correlate with the risk of developing depression. The current thinking suggests that depression in MS is related to immunopathologic mechanisms. The treatment for depression in this population should include psychotherapeutic interventions that focus on the meaning of progression or relapses of the disease in the lives of these patients, as well as other psychosocial issues. Group therapy and cognitive behavioral therapy have been shown to be effective in patients with MS who have depression. Medications, such as desipramine, SSRIs, and others, have been effective as well. Desipramine has been used as a first-line drug in depression in MS because the anticholinergic properties also improve bladder function in these patients.

Pathologic emotionality, as previously discussed in patients with stroke, also can be seen in patients with MS as well as in patients who have other neurologic disorders. The patients can have no control over this disinhibition of emotional expression. Low-dose amitriptyline has been used effectively [(10 mg b.i.d. or three times a day (t.i.d.)] in this syndrome, as have the SSRI medications. Bipolar disorder has been shown to be more prevalent in patients with MS than in the general population (10% vs. 1%). Exactly why this is so is not yet really known. The treatment is just like other bipolar disorders, using mood stabilizers. If the mania is secondary to the steroids that are used to treat the neurologic features of this disorder, a brief course of antipsychotics can be used without mood stabilizers. There is also some form of euphoria in patients with MS that is not quite like mania, which tends to occur in patients with diffuse cerebral disease. These patients have unwavering optimism that is not justified by their current conditions. This does not have to be treated.

LIAISON POTENTIAL

1. The consultation-liaison (C-L) psychiatrist can become attached to the neurology team and make rounds on acute hospitalized patients.
2. The C-L psychiatrist is often welcome and is needed to work in specialty outpatient clinics or with patient organizations, such as MS, PD, or poststroke groups. In these settings, there can be the opportunity to give lectures, see patients on site, or run groups.

Psychiatric Aspects of Surgery and Transplantation

Many of the issues which the C-L psychiatrists will encounter in the surgical setting are covered in various chapters of this book and can be quickly found by looking at the index. Topics which will be particularly pertinent are: delirium, pain, capacity, death and dying, factitious disorders, burn, trauma and psychooncology. These are covered in the chapters appropriate to the subject.

PSYCHOTROPIC MEDICATION

Drug interactions are always important, especially when the patient has medical complications. Decisions often have to be made whether to take a patient off psychotropic medication during a hospitalization for a surgical procedure. If there is an ample time frame, medication can be tapered to avoid withdrawal or discontinuation syndrome. Depending on the surgery, there may be a prolonged period of NPO where only certain medications can be given parentally. A medication such as lithium carbonate is known to fluctuate to potentially toxic levels when there are electrolyte changes or fluid imbalance that can occur during surgery and in the postoperative period. Therefore, a cessation of lithium during this time is often prudent. We have seen our surgical colleagues become upset when it is recommended that a bipolar patient be taken off lithium or other mood stabilizers because of their fear that there will be a "manic episode" in the postoperative period. It is usually easier to deal with the development of manic behavior than it is to face potential renal failure due to lithium toxicity.

It has been shown that patients on selective serotonin reuptake inhibitor (SSRI) antidepressants can have increased intraoperative blood loss and have an increased chance of requiring blood transfusions which is not observed with other antidepressant medications.

When emergency surgery is required, there is often not enough time to consider whether psychotropic drugs should be tapered. In such cases, there can be a drug withdrawal syndrome from medications such as benzodiazepine or opiates or discontinuation syndrome from SSRIs. In cases of alcoholism, there can be alcohol withdrawal syndrome and even delirium tremens (DTs). The consultant needs to be alert because sometimes the general anesthesia, benzodiazepine, and/or narcotics given as part of the postoperative care will mask symptoms due to the abrupt cessation of medication or alcohol.

PREOPERATIVE PHASE

Psychiatric consultants are often requested to evaluate the patient's capacity to give permission for surgery (see

Chapter 15). Delirium, dementia, psychosis, severe depression, and anxiety are the most common reasons for such a request. Preoperative anxiety especially in children is often treated with benzodiazepine. Surgeons frequently will not want to operate on a patient who is very depressed and firmly believe that he or she will not survive the surgery, although we do not know of any evidence-based research which supports this concern. If a patient's psychiatric condition can be put into remission without jeopardizing the patient's physical health, it is usually preferable to institute psychiatric treatment for the patient before surgery.

Sometimes the patient's concern may be related to fear and anxiety about not surviving the surgery or not coming out of anesthesia. Surgery especially with general anesthesia can always be experienced as a life-threatening situation. The following case illustrates one unexpected complication of this reality.

CASE VIGNETTE: "THE MAN WITH NO VOICE"

A 56-year-old man was scheduled to undergo bypass cardiac surgery. On the day before surgery, he totally lost his voice although there were no physical abnormalities for this symptom. He has no previous psychiatric history. He was married with two children and appeared to have a very good relationship with his wife, who was very supportive. He understood that he needed the surgery and was very cooperative but had no idea why he lost his voice. There was no evidence of depression, psychosis, or any indication of conflict. The patient communicated by writing. An exploratory session by the consultant revealed no psychological factors for the loss of voice. The psychiatrist then tested the patient for hypnotizability by the Spiegel roll technique and found that he was +4 (highly hypnotizable). The patient agreed to be hypnotized and easily went into a deep trance. He was then asked once again to express his feelings about the surgery while in the trance. At first, he was communicating by mouthing words but he began to cry. His voice then returned while in the trance. He said he could not bear to say goodbye to his wife and believed that she could not handle things without him. Subsequently after the hypnosis he had two sessions with the psychiatrist, further discussing the subject and his voice gradually returned from a whisper to a normal voice.

INTRAOPERATIVE AWARENESS

There is a phenomenon of intraoperative awareness where the patient will subsequently report some awareness of what happened during the surgery, perhaps remembering music that was played in the operating room during the surgery. In extreme cases, the patient may actually become conscious during the surgery in which case he or she could experience being totally paralyzed and possibly in severe pain. The latter situation is extremely rare and any type of intraoperative awareness is estimated at between 0.5% and 2%. Sequelae of intraoperative awareness can be flashbacks, nightmares, and other symptoms of posttraumatic stress. This would warrant treatment if they persist.

POSTOPERATIVE PHASE

Delirium is one of the most common postoperative problems that consultant psychiatrists address following surgery (this is discussed in another chapter). Frequently the request may be to see the patient for depression but it will turn out that the patient has a delirium.

Pain control is another issue that triggers a request for a psychiatric consultation after surgery (this is also addressed in another chapter). It is important to recognize that the patient may not initially complain of pain and it may be necessary to inquire how severe the postoperative pain is. Patients may also feel that they should avoid any medication for pain because they are afraid that they would become addicted. In such situations, the patient needs to be reassured that this will not happen if the pain medication is taken under proper supervision and if it is tapered during the recovery period.

Any type of surgery has the potential to make the patient feel disfigured and mutilated. Surgery can lead to the loss of function, poor body image, and severe or diminished feelings of self-worth. Pelvic surgery, prostatectomy, osteotomy, throat surgery, and mastectomy are particularly known to create psychosocial stresses and at times result in significant depression. When called to see patients after surgery, other than symptomatic treatment support and assessment for suicidal potential, the best intervention can be a sensitive referral for outpatient follow-up. This needs to be done in a manner so the patient does not feel that the consultant is suggesting that they are now additionally psychologically defective.

Rather, the consultant needs to convey that many people have emotional reactions after surgery and the psychological follow-up can be very helpful as part of the recovery from surgery.

FACTITIOUS DISORDERS

Patients with a factitious disorder have been known to provide a factitious history and/or simulate a medical illness, which can lead to surgery or even multiple surgeries. Such patients may also take advantage of an existing illness and/or interfere with a healing wound perhaps by introducing contaminated material or refracturing a bone leading to still another surgical procedure. Such patients often present with numerous surgical scars and the so-called railroad track or checkerboard abdomen (see Chapter 13 for discussion of factitious disorders).

CARDIAC SURGERY

The time period between first onset of cardiac symptoms and the recommendation for cardiac surgery may be literally only a few weeks or days and sometimes even less than that. Because of the time urgency involved, it is unusual for psychiatrists to be consulted in these situations, even when the patient is highly anxious or depressed. In some cases, however, especially when there is unusual denial or resistance to life-saving surgery, you may be called. In these situations, we often have found that even patients with intense fears may not discuss them, unless invited to do so. This is a good time to teach relaxation exercises, meditation, self-hypnosis, and other types of stress management. These techniques will also have value with all types of surgery as the patients deal with anticipatory anxiety.

By the time the patient is a candidate for a cardiac transplant, he or she is most probably on the brink of death. The fear of not getting a transplant can cause anticipatory bereavement, as the patient feels that "time is running out." Supportive psychotherapy and symptomatic treatment may be useful here. Psychiatrists may be asked to be part of the preassessment team. It has been shown that good coping skills and social support, as well as good pretransplant compliance with treatment regimes are the best predictors of survival.

Therefore, it is important that you assess for the presence of mood syndromes, family adjustment problems, substance abuse, personality disorders, and a history of treatment non-compliance in pretransplant patients. Such knowledge will be useful in planning for posttransplant care. Be careful, however, not to be drawn into situations in which you are asked to decide whether or not a patient will get a transplant (and therefore live or die), based on a psychiatric diagnosis. It is important not to appear like a policeman so that you can gain the trust of the patient. You should focus instead on making an objective psychiatric evaluation that takes into consideration the patient's social supports, motivation, and understanding, as well as the potential for compliance with the complicated posttransplant regimen. One can prevent being drawn into being the gatekeeper if the transplant team has scientifically valid data-based criteria for exclusion on which to base the team decision.

There are a number of other issues specific to cardiac transplant patients about which you may be called to consult. The family members of posttransplant patients often feel great emotional upheaval and may require psychological support. Whatever you can do to minimize the negative effects of the transplant experience on the family caregiver will indirectly help the patient as well. Symptoms of post-traumatic stress disorder (PTSD) are a complication for some heart transplant patients. Use of immunosuppressants, such as steroids and antirejection medications (i.e., cyclosporin), may lead to delirium, depression, and psychotic manifestations (e.g., delusions and auditory and visual hallucinations).

Keep in mind that the patient realizes that he or she is surviving only because somebody else has died and that he or she now has that person's heart. There is often survivor guilt, as well as identification with the donor, whether or not the recipient actually knows about the donor. The recipient may want to meet the family of the donor and even establish a relationship with them.

Postoperative Delirium After Cardiac Surgery

There appears to be a greater risk of delirium in cardiac surgery than in other types of surgery. This may be related to the time spent on extracorporeal circulation. You may be called to help in the management of these patients. You should always consider the possibility of all the usual causes of delirium, including, but not limited to, cerebrovascular events (e.g., emboli, sepsis, drug side effects and interactions, and metabolic changes). Medications used for pain control, particularly meperidine, can be the culprit, and switching to an alternate pain control drug, such as morphine, may be helpful. In postcardiotomy patients, a specific etiology for the delirium may not be evident. Nevertheless, symptomatic treatment of delirium should be instituted (see Chapter 10).

CASE VIGNETTE: CONFUSED AFTER OPEN HEART SURGERY

A successful 70-year-old business executive was diagnosed as needing coronary artery bypass graft (CABG) surgery. He had two grafts performed in open-heart bypass surgery without any complications. In the second day post surgery, he became acutely agitated, pulling out lines, and acting in a paranoid manner. There were no localizing symptoms, and psychiatric consultation was called. The patient was diagnosed as having an acute onset of delirium. He was given haloperidol intravenously (IV), and surgery staff was advised to look into possible organic etiology for the delirium. The patient was determined to have previously undiagnosed diabetic hyperglycemia. As his symptoms began to resolve, he was switched to risperidone, which was discontinued before discharge.

AMPUTATION

Surgical amputation can be necessary because of trauma or because of diseases such as diabetes and cancer.

No matter what the cause, an amputation represents a unique assault on the patient's integrity and sense of wholeness. How the psychological and social consequences of the amputation are handled is just as important as the healing of the stump itself.

We have noted that a few days after an amputation, patients frequently will show a very good outward facade. They seem to be happy and talk about looking forward to rehabilitation treatment. The novice consultant erroneously may believe that the patient is doing well and does not need any follow up. In reality, what is most likely being seen is denial, and such patients are still quite vulnerable to becoming severely depressed.

142 Psychosomatic Medicine: A Practical Guide

Phantom phenomena—Phantom phenomena refers to the patient experiencing the amputated limb as still being present and is a universal consequence of amputation. Phantom pain is experienced as painful sensations, which are felt in the stump of a phantom limb. The patient feels as if the absent limb is still present and is causing extreme pain. At least 80% of patients will experience phantom pain. One common theory to explain these sensations is that a cortical representation of the missing limb is created in the brain.

Grief response—After an initial period of denial, the amputee usually goes through a period of anger. Because one cannot easily be angry at something that does not exist, the anger is likely to be displaced onto others or the self. The intense grief response is similar to the experience of losing a loved one. However, the patient is not only grieving the lost limb, but also is grieving his or her former self-image.

As the patient moves past this stage, he or she may become preoccupied with a new prosthesis. There can be unrealistic expectations about the prosthesis, which can lead to disappointments for patients and families. Living with a prosthesis can cause social isolation, which, in turn, can cause or intensify depressive symptoms. Nightmares and flashbacks are common after amputation and will usually diminish with time and frequency of episodes. Grunert et al. described three type of flashbacks that had prognostic significance:

1. Replay—A replaying of the events immediately preceding the accident and continuing until the time of injury (more than 90% of patients replaying events returned to employment).
2. Appraisal—An image of the injured hand immediately after the replay.
3. Projected—An image of injuries worse than the real injury. (Those patients with a combination of the latter two types were least likely to return to work.)

Replantation—There is increasing surgical experience with replantation of severed fingers, toes, limbs, and male genitalia after traumatic injuries. As illustrated in the following vignette, the psychological state before the accident will influence the emotional state post replantation.

CASE VIGNETTE: ACCEPTING RESPONSIBILITY

A 24-year-old man was returning from a fight with his girl-friend. He was in a preoccupied state and drove carelessly around a wet corner. He lost his right arm in the subsequent accident and had the limb successfully replanted. He contin-ues to blame his girlfriend for the injury. Issues of accepting responsibility became the major focus of his rehabilitation and his failure to recover function in the limb. Only after he had therapy to help him work through his state of "learned helplessness" was the patient able to progress to a better recovery.

The same psychological issues described in the burn and trauma patient are relevant after a replantation. Flashbacks can be particularly graphic because there is a focus on the idea of mutilation. There will be increased anxiety specifically about the physical survival of the reattached limb. Some-times leeches are attached that can promote blood flow from the engorged extremity and this can cause a psychological response. The staff may tell the patient that their bluish swollen, functionless limb is "doing great," but the patient is more likely terrified about losing the limb again. Therapeutic intervention may give the patient a chance to verbalize these fears and deal with anticipatory anxiety about the loss.

TRANSPLANTATION SURGERY

Cardiac, liver, and renal transplantations are mentioned else-where in this book. Lung, pancreatic, and bone marrow transplants are also being done on a regular basis at many medical centers. More recently brain tissue, limb transplanta-tion, and facial transplant have been done to a limited degree.

Transplants can come from a living donor, that is, kidney, partial liver or bone marrow, or can be cadaveric. Rarely there are the so-called domino transplants where multiple sequen-tial procedures are done. For example, a liver in one person produces abnormal harmful proteins but functions well in another person. So it is retransplanted in another person while that donor receives a living or cadaveric transplant. In other cases, a heart lung transplant is performed in a patient who has a normal heart but the chance of success is better if both organs are transplanted. Therefore, the normal heart goes to another patient. Still other situations involve willing living donors of kidneys who are not compatible with their loved ones but are comparable with a third person. Therefore, multiple procedures can be done sequentially or at the same time.

Each type of transplant situation presents its own specific issues and concurrent psychosocial factors and conflicts. The psychiatrist is often part of the transplant team and needs to understand the psychological factors involved frequently after transplant from a living person. The main attention is focused on the recipient with great jubilation if it appears to be successful. This can leave the donor who is in fact the "hero" feeling neglected. If the transplant fails, the donor and the recipient may feel great loss and guilt. Psychological follow-up in such situations can be helpful.

There is often high anxiety during the waiting period for the transplant patient, as the patient is not only concerned for his or her health and life but also worried if he or she will be high enough on the list to get the next transplant. At times, there are complicated family dynamics as family members are asked to be tested to determine if they are a compatible match for a donation.

In cases of cadaveric transplant, the recipient is in a situation of hoping that some anonymous person will die so he or she can get a transplant. Some patients want to meet the family of the cadaveric donor and some families of donors want to meet the recipient. There will be different local guidelines to follow as well as the dictates of the clinical situation. Some patients have stated that they believe that they have taken on some of the characteristics of the donor. There is no validity to such a possibility but the psychological issues here may have to be evaluated.

SELECTION FOR TRANSPLANT

Psychosocial factors are usually included in the selection criteria for transplantation and a psychiatrist or other mental health professional is often part of the transplant team. There are also scales such as the Transplant Evaluation Reading Scale (TERS) and the Psychosocial Assessments of Candidates for Transplant Scale (PACTS). There is variability depending on the organ, hospital, clinical setting, and individual clinical situation as to whether or not psychological data should be used as a determining factor in determining the place on the transplant list or whether a patient should receive a transplant. There is disagreement whether or not adherence to posttransplant medication and treatment plan can be predicted even by pretransplant behavior such as compliance to dialysis or abstaining from alcohol intake. In the posttransplant period, the psychiatrist needs to be alert about drug interaction between any psychotropic medication and the latest immunosuppressant drug that are being used. As the frontiers for transplant surgery are further advanced so will be the challenges to the C-L psychiatrist. The medical and pharmacologic issues will become more complicated, so will the psychological meaning and the impact of the transplantation as well as the psychological adjustment. This will call for new psychological understanding and psychotherapeutic techniques.

LIAISON POTENTIAL

1. Specialized surgery programs will sometimes include psychiatrists as part of their team approach. This is common in burn and trauma units. Other surgical teams such as bariatric surgery for obesity, cancer surgery teams especially for mastectomies and radical ear, nose, and throat (ENT) surgery particularly after laryngectomies are known for using psychiatrists with liaison approach.
2. Special situations in surgery are known to frequently bring with them complex psychiatric issues. If psychiatrists have a working relationship with the surgeon, they may become involved in the planning of unusual surgical situations. Examples might include amputation, reimplantation, separation of conjoint twins, eye or ear surgery resulting in blindness or loss of hearing or conversely in restoration of these senses, facial transplants, and "domino" transplantation situations.
3. Psychiatrists can be assigned to various transplant teams in a liaison role. In such situations, they may evaluate all recipients and donors when feasible. This will also put them in better position to evaluate postoperative psychiatric issues.

12 Human Immunodeficiency Virus/Acquired Immunodeficiency Syndrome Psychiatry

---

Essential Concepts

Human immunodeficiency virus (HIV) syndrome is a dynamic entity, so you should update yourself continuously on developments in diagnosis and treatment.

- HIV-infected patients are very sensitive to medications, particularly to the side effects of drugs that affect the central nervous system. Therefore, the dictum "start low and go slow" applies whenever you are treating HIV-infected individuals.
- HIV and acquired immunodeficiency syndrome (AIDS) patients are often on multiple medications. It is imperative for you to know what they are, as they may interact with medications that you are prescribing. In addition, these medications also have neuropsychiatric manifestations.
- You should not dismiss depressive symptoms as "normal" consequences of being diagnosed with a terminal illness. A complete evaluation and adequate treatment are always warranted.

With the advent of highly active antiretroviral therapy (HAART) or what is now known as combination antiretroviral therapy (CART), the death rates from AIDS have decreased. However, the prevalence of HIV continues to increase and recent HIV surveillance data reveal that the increase is found in young males who have sex with men. More people are living longer and so some people are engaging in more risky behavior.

The most recent Centers for Disease Control and Prevention (CDC) AIDS surveillance data revised in June 2007 show that there were 41,987 estimated AIDS cases in 2005 up from 40,655 cases in 2004 with a cumulative total of 984,115 cases of AIDS in the United States in 2005. Our understanding of the HIV epidemic has come a long way from the days when only gay white males were considered vulnerable to the disease. The faces of HIV are not only the gay men or the intravenous (IV) drug abusers; they now also include the older, so-called geriatric age-group and women. HIV has infected, and continues to infect, men, women, and children of many different age-groups, ethnicities, sexual preferences, socioeconomic classes, and cultural backgrounds. In addition to the medical complications to which HIV-infected individuals are susceptible, the disease can cause a range of psychiatric problems. For this reason, it is quite common to encounter these patients in the consultation-liaison (C-L) setting.

THE RELATIONSHIP BETWEEN PSYCHIATRIC DISORDERS AND HUMAN IMMUNODEFICIENCY VIRUS

Psychiatric disorders interface with HIV in various ways.

1. There are patients with premorbid psychiatric disorders (e.g., major affective disorder, schizophrenia, and substance abuse) that existed before being infected.
2. There are patients who are impacted by real-life events (e.g., loss of job, death of a parent, etc.) that are unrelated to HIV infection.
3. There are psychiatric phenomena secondary to medical conditions (e.g., delirium secondary to sepsis and dementia secondary to medical causes) that are characteristic of patients with AIDS.

There are certain points in the course of HIV infection when patients are more vulnerable to developing psychiatric disorders:

1. *At seroconversion*. Finding out about their status can cause severe anxiety, depression, brief psychotic disorder, acute

stress disorder, or a post-traumatic stress disorder (PTSD)-like syndrome, among others.

2. *During the adaptation to an essentially asymptomatic period.* The patient who is HIV positive (but asymptomatic) feels very anxious and is very vigilant about any body lesions and other physical symptoms.

3. *During the transition to symptomatic disease.* When patients begin to develop opportunistic infections, they can develop psychiatric disorders from the disease process itself, medications used to treat the complications of HIV, and emotional reactions to the disease.

4. *When patients develop frank AIDS.* One of the most common psychiatric complications of AIDS is delirium, which is seen often when patients develop full-blown AIDS. Another common psychiatric syndrome during this stage is HIV-associated dementia (HAD).

5. *When CD4 and viral load levels fluctuate.* Anxiety and depression often accompany patients' reactions to decreased CD4 cell counts and increased viral loads.

6. *When patients are on CART drugs.* The CART drugs themselves cause neuropsychiatric side effects. Moreover, there are psychological issues that are related to coping with taking these medications.

Psychiatric conditions that are seen in HIV/AIDS are shown in Table 12.1. One of your most important tasks in treating these patients is to identify whether or not a psychiatric condition is secondary to medical etiology (e.g., due to medications, brain lymphoma, etc.). If a condition will resolve as a result of

TABLE 12.1. Psychiatric Disorders in Human Immunodeficiency Virus

Depressive disorders
Anxiety disorders
Substance use disorders
Cognitive disorders
Pain syndromes
Adjustment disorders
Sleep disorders
Sexual disorders
Manic disorders
Psychotic disorders
Personality disorders

a medical intervention, it may make using psychotropic drug use unnecessary.

PSYCHOLOGICAL CONSEQUENCES OF SEROCONVERSION

Once an individual is diagnosed with HIV, he or she goes through stages quite similar to those previously described in dealing with death and cancer. During the initial crisis, the patient has intense emotions. He or she is in shock, quite angry, afraid, and often denial is quite strong. It is not uncommon for a patient to disbelieve the initial diagnosis and to request repeat testing and second opinions. These patients may not be able to grasp and understand what is being relayed to them. When denial wanes, the patient becomes distressed and angry. Guilt, self-pity, depression, and acting out replace the denial in this transitional stage. Common dysfunctional responses include, "I'm going to die anyway, so I'll just continue to use drugs and be happy" or "If I'm infected, then I'll infect others too." Once patients reach the stage of acceptance, they often develop a fighting spirit and may become activists for HIV causes. They may become quite active in finding out what new advances there are, where drug studies are being done, and what alternative options are available to them. There can be a preparatory stage where patients actually start to plan their funerals and memorial services and they may compose their own epitaphs. They may try to reunite with estranged loved ones, write their living wills, and appoint health care proxies. It is important to remember that there is no definitive separation between stages. They may overlap or, in some cases, not be found.

DEPRESSION AND HUMAN IMMUNODEFICIENCY VIRUS

Major depression is among the most common psychiatric disorders in HIV. It is seen in up to 30% of patients in some studies. Depressive symptoms are quite common, but, once again, it must be emphasized that you should not dismiss these symptoms as "normal." A thorough evaluation is essential. Recognize that a number of the symptoms of depression can be confused with medical problems, which can lead to a potential false diagnosis of depression. We suggest that you place more emphasis on the cognitive symptoms of depression (e.g., hopelessness, helplessness, guilt, anhedonia, etc.) more than the neurovegetative symptoms (e.g., sleep, appetite, and energy disturbances, etc.) to make a diagnosis of clinical depression in AIDS patients.

Treatment of Depression

All antidepressants appear equally effective in AIDS patients. In general, we have found that HIV patients respond more quickly and at lower doses than non-HIV patients. Because patients with HIV/AIDS are usually on multiple medications, drug interactions with antidepressants are especially likely. AIDS patients are particularly sensitive to the side effects of psychotropic drugs, and, for this reason, selective serotonin reuptake inhibitors (SSRIs) have largely supplanted tricyclic antidepressants (TCAs) as first-line antidepressants for this population. Psychostimulants can be very useful, particularly in the severely medically ill, but avoid them if your patient is psychotic.

SUICIDE AND HUMAN IMMUNODEFICIENCY VIRUS

CASE VIGNETTE: THE EXPIRED PHENOBARBITALS

Gerry is a 34-year-old HIV-positive white gay male who, with his partner, went to see a physician who was well known for his views regarding euthanasia. Gerry and his lover were newly diagnosed with HIV and, in those days, there was only azidothymidine (AZT). They asked for and got enough phenobarbital prescriptions to kill themselves. They were convinced that they would rather die than suffer the consequences of HIV. Gerry's partner went ahead and took the pills and died, but Gerry demurred. He kept the pills in his drawer and brought them with him when he moved to the East coast a year later. He felt he needed to feel he could control his life. Three years later, Gerry still had the pills and finally got rid of them, with the help of his therapist.

Suicidality in AIDS patients is a complicated issue. Requests for assisted suicide and euthanasia may be seen as rational, but they deserve a serious evaluation to rule out a treatable psychiatric condition. Research has shown varying rates among different groups, with AIDS patients having lower suicide rates than those with only HIV. Be watchful of the patient who decides to discontinue treatment for potentially treatable complications; this can possibly be a passive suicidal gesture.

ANXIETY AND HUMAN IMMUNODEFICIENCY VIRUS

As you might expect, anxiety is quite common in HIV patients. At the time of initial diagnosis, anxiety about the future is most salient. Physical symptoms that would have otherwise been dismissed now assume a significance that causes more anxiety and fear. Many patients try to conceal their HIV status, sexual orientation, illicit drug use, and the medications they are taking, all of which adds to their anxiety. A PTSD-like syndrome has been reported in patients upon learning of their seroconversion as well as in others who have suffered multiple losses from AIDS. You will see the entire spectrum of anxiety disorders, from adjustment disorder to panic disorder with agoraphobia, in this population. Recall that anxiety can present as somatic symptoms and therefore may be difficult to differentiate from symptoms of medical illness.

Treatment of Anxiety

After having done a thorough evaluation to rule out possible organic causes, including substance use, you can treat anxiety using either pharmacologic or nonpharmacologic modalities. Among medications, benzodiazepines are usually first line, especially in cases where the anxiety is time limited. Be judicious with benzodiazepines when treating patients with substance use histories. For more chronic anxiety, we suggest either SSRIs or buspirone. Nonpharmacologic techniques include meditation, muscle relaxation, biofeedback, hypnosis, imagery, acupuncture, and individual or group psychotherapy.

PSYCHOTIC DISORDERS IN HUMAN IMMUNODEFICIENCY VIRUS

The prevalence of psychosis in HIV-infected individuals is highly variable. It is also important to include in the differential diagnosis the possibility that the psychosis is secondary to a treatable medical condition. Psychosis in HIV can be due to several factors: opportunistic infections; the direct effects of HIV in the brain; a side effect of medications and other medical/surgical treatments; or a symptom of substance abuse, intoxication, withdrawal, or conventional psychiatric disorders, such as schizophrenia and bipolar disorder.

Treatment of Psychotic Disorders

Once again, when treating HIV-infected individuals, the dictum, "start low and go slow" applies. In particular, these patients are quite sensitive to the extrapyramidal and anticholinergic side effects of antipsychotic drugs. We recommend using haloperidol in very low doses, newer atypical antipsychotics (risperidone, olanzapine, and quetiapine), or molindone.

COGNITIVE DISORDERS AND HUMAN IMMUNODEFICIENCY VIRUS

Cognitive disorders in HIV are commonly one of two syndromes: minor cognitive motor disorder and HIV Associated Dementia (HAD).

Minor cognitive motor disorder is diagnosed if any two of the following are present:

1. Impaired attention/concentration
2. Mental slowing
3. Impaired memory
4. Slowed movements
5. Impaired coordination
6. Personality change/irritability/lability

In addition, these symptoms are verified by neurologic examination (e.g., hyperreflexia, saccadic eye movements, frontal release signs, and ataxia); functional impairment is less than that required for dementia and there is no other etiology. HIV-infected individuals present with varying manifestations of HAD. This is usually associated with the later stages of the disease, although it may occur as the AIDS-defining condition with patients who are not yet severely immunocompromised. There are specific risk factors associated with HAD and these include older age at diagnosis, wasting syndrome, anemia, and substance use history. The dementia that is found in HIV-infected individuals is similar to the subcortical dementias that are seen in Parkinson's or Wilson's disease. With the introduction of potent antiretroviral therapy drug combinations that include drugs that penetrate the blood–brain barrier, the incidence of HAD has decreased. In patients who have been diagnosed with HAD, treatment with CART, particularly combinations that include AZT or abacavir, has caused, at the very least, a partial improvement of cognitive deficits.

Early HAD is often difficult to recognize and differentiate from depression. Symptoms can include the following:

1. Apathy
2. Slowed information processing
3. Unsteady gait or dyscoordination
4. Difficulty with formerly automatic tasks
5. Forgetfulness
6. Mild tremors
7. Visuoconstructive deficits

In late HAD, the symptoms can include the following:

1. Psychotic features
2. Severe attention deficit
3. Severe memory loss
4. Personality changes: irritability, mania
5. Ataxia
6. Prominent tremors
7. Mutism, delusions, and hallucinations

As mentioned earlier, HIV dementia appears to improve when patients are on CART. In addition, symptomatic treatment can consist of using low doses of neuroleptics, if psychotic, manic, or agitated features are present. Antidepressants can be used in depression and antianxiety agents can be used for anxiety. Supportive treatment includes reminder systems (e.g., notebooks, signs, diaries, alarms, etc.), speaking to these patients simply and slowly and reorienting them, and so forth.

PAIN SYNDROMES AND HUMAN IMMUNODEFICIENCY VIRUS

The topic of pain syndromes (and HIV) is presented in Chapter 14. This also applies to pain in HIV/AIDS. However, it is useful to remember that HIV/AIDS patients with pain are often undertreated and underdiagnosed. The prevalence of pain in these patients can be as high as 30–80%. The causes are usually multifactorial. Pain in HIV/AIDS can be a consequence of HIV related conditions, a side effect of HIV/AIDS therapies or not at all related to HIV/AIDS.

SPECIAL ISSUES IN HIGHLY ACTIVE ANTIRETROVIRAL THERAPY

CASE VIGNETTE: THE SO-CALLED NEW LIFE WITH CART

Elizabeth had several hospitalizations after being diagnosed with HIV in 1985. She had looked quite sick and had been on disability for many years. She also has not used drugs for the last 15 years. Since starting the new "cocktail" regimens for HIV, however, she had not been hospitalized, had gained weight, and no longer looked "sick" at all. She felt energized and ready to relive her life again. The harsh reality of "living" dashed all of her hopes. She has been unable to find a job that would give her benefits so she can continue her medications. Most jobs that were available to her would disqualify her for drug assistance, but the benefits would not allow her to have her medications. She decided to continue to be unemployed. Life became quite boring for her because she was healthier and had a lot of time on her hands. She then started using drugs again and was soon back on the same road she had traveled before she contracted AIDS.

More new HIV drugs and drug classes are being discovered as the years pass. At the time of this writing, the classes include nucleoside/nucleotide reverse transcriptase inhibitors, nonnucleoside reverse transcriptase inhibitors, protease inhibitors, entry inhibitors and more recently, integrase inhibitors. In addition, there are the dual-class fixed-dose combinations that were created to improve adherence and simplify treatment regimens. It is important for the psychiatrist to know what medications the patient is on. First and foremost is the need to be aware of drug–drug interactions. Although most of these are essentially seen *in vitro*, it still is our responsibility to be cautious and informed. The most common interactions to watch are those between ritonavir (Norvir) and benzodiazepines and hypnotics. Clozapine and pimozide are contraindicated when using CART. Caution should be exercised when using bupropion with protease inhibitors as well. In addition, the use of CART has brought chronic side effects that can be demoralizing and can lead to depression. These include metabolic abnormalities, gastrointestinal (GI) side effects, and lipodystrophy, among others. Another reality is that HIV/AIDS patients are living longer; therefore, they are more vulnerable to psychological problems that are associated with living with chronic disease, such as stigma, financial issues, and the difficult battle against the temptation of drug use. Now, more than ever, psychiatric care is an essential part of the multidisciplinary treatment of patients with HIV/AIDS.

LIAISON POTENTIAL

The role of psychiatrists in the field of HIV/AIDS has become more relevant because patients with HIV have been living longer. This has allowed C-L psychiatrists to do various types of liaison work that is related to AIDS. Examples of such activities are:

1. Participate in lectures and education programs in schools, health centers, as well as for high-risk groups, such as drug programs, and with gay groups.
2. Lecture medical students, residents, and nurses about the psychiatric aspects of AIDS and related issues (e.g., stigma, high-risk factors, and adherence).
3. Design and participate in activities, such as AIDS Memorial Service, AIDS Quilting Program, groups to prevent burnout, and so on.
4. Attend regular medical rounds with the AIDS medical team.
5. Participate and take leadership role with AIDS psychosocial team that often consists of social workers, case managers, HIV counselors, clinical nurse specialists, and psychologists.
6. See patient for psychiatric care at the site of HIV medical clinics.

Somatoform Disorders, Factitious Disorders, and Malingering

> ### Essential Concepts
> - If signs and symptoms do not follow physiologically expected mechanisms, somatization must be in the differential diagnosis.
> - Somatization may coexist with any physical illness and initially may mask the illness.
> - Abrupt changes in personality, mood, and ability to function, as well as rapid fluctuations in mental status suggest that a physical diagnosis is more likely.
> - Secondary gain strongly suggests either malingering or factitious disorder, *but* the absence of secondary gain does not rule out some other cause.
> - Every patient is entitled to at least one good medical workup.

There is no other area of medicine where the mind–body relationship assumes a more significant role than in the field of somatization where the lines blur between medicine and psychiatry. The medical training of the consultation-liaison (C-L) psychiatrist becomes crucial. Patients present with various physical problems when, in reality, the predominant problem is psychological. It is the task of the C-L psychiatrist to deal with the true nature of the problem and to understand the defenses that are used by patients to avoid dealing with their psychological issues. Somatization is better conceptualized as a symptom that can be found in various disorders that are classified under the main category of somatoform disorders, but it is also seen in the category of factitious disorders. Somatization also has its costs. Somatizers cost the health care system much more than nonsomatizers in terms of total charges, physician visits, and hospital charges. It also affects productivity, in that somatizers are sick and out of work a lot more often than the general population. It is often a very difficult task for the psychiatrist to overtly make this diagnosis, particularly because he or she has to balance the stigma attached to the label of "somatizing" with the possibility that something is truly wrong in the physical sense and needs to be attended to or else a serious medical problem may be missed.

PATHOPHYSIOLOGICAL MECHANISMS

Patients with somatoform disorders actually feel what they say they feel. There are several pathophysiologic pathways that bring this about. These include physiological mechanisms, such as autonomic arousal, muscle tension, hyperventilation, physiological effects of inactivity, sleep disturbances, and cerebral information processing. Among the psychological mechanisms involved are mood, beliefs, perceptual factors, and personality factors. Other mechanisms, such as the disability system, the health care system, and the reinforcing actions of friends and relatives also foster the development of somatization. It is necessary to be able to distinguish the differences between somatoform disorders and factitious disorders where somatization is the prominent symptom. Two essential factors to consider are the voluntary nature of the production of symptoms and the presence of secondary gain (e.g., attention, avoidance of unpleasant tasks, material rewards, disability, "3 hots and a cot," etc.). Production of somatic symptoms in *factitious disorders* and *malingering* is voluntary, whereas it is involuntary in *somatoform disorders*. There is an unconscious gain that is noted in somatoform disorders and factitious disorders, whereas it is conscious in malingering.

SOMATOFORM DISORDERS

This is a group of disorders in which patients present with physical symptoms for which an adequate medical explanation cannot be found. Somatoform disorders are not the result of conscious malingering or factitious disorders. The diagnosis of somatoform disorder implies that psychological factors contribute to the nature of the symptoms, onset, severity, and duration. They include the following, which are under the category of "somatoform disorder" [as listed in Diagnostic and Statistical Manual of Mental Disorders, Fourth Edition (DSM-IV)]:

- Somatization disorder
- Conversion disorder
- Hypochondriasis
- Body dysmorphic disorder
- Somatoform pain disorder
- Undifferentiated somatoform disorder
- Somatoform disorder, not otherwise specified (NOS)

Somatization Disorder

Somatization disorder is known to most as "hysteria" and recalls the famous painting by Charcot of a woman fainting. The hysteric also has been stereotyped as a young woman who is quite suggestible; however, modern psychiatry has broadened this definition. Although more predominantly found in women (ratio 10:1), this condition also exists in men. The characteristic finding is a multiplicity of symptoms that involve multiple organ systems [typically described by the mnemonic FOOT: Four gastrointestinal (GI) symptoms, One pseudoneurologic symptom, One sexual symptom, and Two pain symptoms]. Somatization disorder is usually a chronic condition, whose onset is usually before the age of 30 years. More importantly, patients with this condition have excessive medical help-seeking behavior.

The symptoms of somatization can be interpreted in various ways: as a means to express the patient's emotions, as a symbolic manifestation of a feeling or belief, or as a way to avoid obligations. Treatment consists of giving a psychophysiological explanation for the symptoms to the patient, allowing for regular, but brief, follow-up visits with the same primary physician (so that the patient does not need to develop new symptoms to get medical attention), and avoiding unnecessary costly interventions. It may be that a sympathetic relationship with a health care provider is the most important aspect of treatment. It has also been shown that patients with this condition who are treated with cognitive behavioral therapy (CBT) by a mental health professional are more likely to show improvement than patients who received standard medical care.

Conversion Disorder

---

*CASE VIGNETTE: PARALYSIS TO CONTROL
SEXUAL IMPULSE*

*A 29-year-old married woman presented to the emergency
room (ER) with inability to walk. At the time, the patient was
staying with her brother-in-law's family while her husband
was in the Gulf War. Workup to establish the etiology of
the apparent paralysis was negative. There were no abnormal
reflexes and no anatomic explanation could be found. The
neurology service then called the C-L psychiatrist who spoke
to the patient at length. The patient recalled that after a
couple of days visiting with her in-laws, she felt anxious
and fearful when walking by her brother-in-law's room. The
patient also admitted to sexual fantasy involving her and her
brother-in-law. The following morning, she was unable to walk.
After treatment using suggestion, coupled with supportive
psychotherapy that focused on her guilt because she was
naturally attracted to others while missing her husband, the
patient walked again.*

Unlike somatization disorder where several symptoms
affect several organ systems, conversion disorder is
monosymptomatic and usually involves the voluntary
nervous system (i.e., motor, of arms and legs; sensory, as
in pain; or special senses, as in vision or hearing). This
is often (but not exclusively) found in young adults and
adolescents, in those with a low intelligence quotient (IQ)
and/or educational attainment, and in those who belong to a
lower socioeconomic group. Conversion disorder also is seen
commonly in military personnel who are exposed to combat.
"La belle indifference" often is used to describe patients with
conversion disorder to highlight the fact that these patients
do not seem perturbed by the fact that they are blind, mute,
paralyzed, and so forth.

The symptoms can be the result of repression of unconscious intrapsychic conflicts and the conversion of the anxiety
into a physical symptom. The symptom often has a symbolic
relation to the unconscious conflict. Treatment may include

the use of suggestion, persuasion, and hypnosis. The patient needs to be in a therapeutic relationship where the therapist is a caring and authoritative person.

Hypochondriasis

CASE VIGNETTE: THIS TIME IT IS A BRAIN TUMOR

A 30-year-old married man presented with a severe headache. The C-L psychiatrist was called when the neurosurgeons could not justify the patient's symptoms with his presentation. Magnetic resonance imaging (MRI) showed no findings. The patient was insistent that he may have a brain tumor and wanted to be given a complete workup to rule this out. Yet, despite showing him the studies that were done, all of which did not show a brain tumor, the patient insisted on a second opinion. After talking to the patient, the psychiatrist found out that he was newly married. The patient admitted to anxieties about his marriage. As it turned out, the patient developed headaches soon after the wedding and had been going to various doctors trying to find out if he had a brain tumor. The patient also had appetite and sleep disturbances that were related to this, as well as feelings of hopelessness and helplessness. He had a history of previously believing he had a heart condition. He required extensive tests before he accepted that this was not the case. The patient was started on a selective serotonin reuptake inhibitor (SSRI) and was engaged in individual and couple therapy. The patient was followed up in the outpatient C-L service and, after a few weeks, began to improve.

Lay people and even health care personnel often talk about this one or that one being a "hypochondriac." We need to be a bit more careful when using this term. Hypochondriasis is a preoccupation with the fear of contracting, or the belief of having, a serious disease. What happens is that there is a misinterpretation of symptoms, and patients may have a comorbid psychiatric condition, such as depression and anxiety. Patients want to get into the "sick role" as a form of escape. The diagnosis is suggested by history and examination. It is confirmed when the symptoms persists more than or equal to 6 months and cannot be attributed to depression or another psychological disorder.

The symptoms can be interpreted as aggressive and hostile wishes toward others that are transformed into physical complaints. This is often used as a defense against guilt. Treatment consists of regularly scheduled physical examinations and documentation of symptoms. It is important to get the needed psychiatric interventions, although these patients are quite resistant to this approach. Brief individual CBT interventions developed specifically to alter and restructure hypochondriacal beliefs appear to have significant beneficial long-term effects on the symptoms of hypochondriasis.

Body Dysmorphic Disorder

Body dysmorphic disorder is a serious illness where a person is preoccupied with a minor or imaginary physical flaw usually of skin, hair, or nose. Males with this condition are more likely to have comorbid substance abuse issues (50%) and females have comorbid anxiety and panic.

CASE VIGNETTE: PREOCCUPATION ABOUT
A CONDITION THAT WAS BARELY THERE

A handsome 20-year-old man, who was a college senior, was seen in consultation because he had infected lesions in the face that required intravenous (IV) antibiotics. Apparently, a few months before, he felt that his acne was so bad that people talked and laughed about him, although objectively it was quite minimal. He felt quite embarrassed by this and, as a consequence, he stayed in his room most of the time and did not socialize or attend any extracurricular activity. He was thinking about the pimples on his face almost all day and could hardly concentrate on his schoolwork. The patient then started picking on the small pimples, eventually infecting them so that they required IV antibiotics. On psychiatric evaluation, it was found that the young man was very anxious about his future after college and had been quite depressed about this. He had the classic symptoms of depression. The patient was treated with an SSRI, as well as CBT and showed improvement after approximately 16 weeks of treatment.

In the last few years, we have seen several patients with body dysmorphia who were referred by plastic surgeons after the patient requested plastic surgery. The most common procedure requested was rhinoplasty. In some of these situations, the patient's nose and facial appearance was noted to be quite attractive. These were mostly women, but this situation can occur in men. More recently, we have seen males in their teens and 20s who were preoccupied with their abdominal muscles, which they felt were below average, when clearly the opposite was true. We also have been called in as consultants for young men who were using steroids to improve their appearance, and some of them may fall in this diagnostic category. Body dysmorphic disorder, sometimes known as *dysmorphophobia*, is a preoccupation with an imagined defect or an exaggerated distortion of a minor defect in physical appearance. There is a high comorbidity, with major depression (90%), anxiety disorder (70%), and psychotic disorder (30%). There is a displacement of a sexual or emotional conflict onto a nonrelated body part. Treatment of the comorbid psychiatric condition is essential. Psychopharmacotherapy, particularly using SSRIs, with individual psychotherapy where there is a good therapeutic alliance, is the treatment of choice. Treatment options include CBT frequently combined with SSRI medication.

Somatoform Pain Disorder

In this particular disorder, the presence of pain is the "predominant focus of clinical attention." Pain is not fully accounted for by a nonpsychiatric medical or neurologic condition. It does not mean, however, that there is no physical reason for the pain. Pain can be associated with only psychological factors or it can be associated with both psychological factors and a general medical condition, according to DSM-IV. The interpretation of the symptoms can be related to the atonement for perceived wrongdoing, the expiation of guilt, or to suppressed aggression. Treatment for this disorder includes pharmacotherapy, CBT, individual psychotherapy, and pain programs.

Nonspecific Somatoform Disorders

These include undifferentiated somatoform disorder, where there are unexplained physical symptoms that last for at least 6 months, and somatoform disorder, NOS, which is a residual category.

FACTITIOUS DISORDERS

DSM-IV classifies factitious disorders differently from somatoform disorders. A factitious disorder is where an individual symptom or symptoms are induced or falsified by the patient. The motivation for the behavior is usually to assume the "sick role." There are no discernible external incentives for the behavior.

CASE VIGNETTE: THE MYSTERIOUS NONHEALING LESION

A consultation was requested by a plastic surgery service for a 38-year-old female nurse who had worked for a dermatologist for many years and now presented to the hospital with a nonhealing ulcerating lesion on the dorsal aspect of her left hand. She was febrile and was not responding to antibiotics as an outpatient. This was the third hospitalization for this lesion. The lesion would heal after a prolonged hospitalization with IV antibiotics and then, after being home briefly, the lesion recurred. Cultures did not reveal unusual organisms and medical workup did not reveal any possible etiology. The C-L psychiatrist focused mainly on establishing a relationship with the patient and encouraging her to talk about her concerns about the lesion. On the third visit, the patient revealed that she was convinced that mites from the ongoing construction work near her house were the cause of the lesion. She claimed that she had even extracted them from the lesion and viewed them under the microscope in the dermatologist's office. She convinced one of the junior house staff to take a look under the laboratory microscope. Several consultants ultimately concluded that there was no infestation. The staff then decided to watch the patient surreptitiously and she was observed to be scraping her wound with an unsterile scalpel and rubbing her unwashed fingers over the lesion. Although she had never previously presented with psychiatric symptoms, shortly after she was noted to be infecting the lesion herself, she developed psychotic symptoms. She became delusional, religiously preoccupied—performing special religious rites to take the "evil spirits" away, as she believed that they had caused her lesions. The patient was then treated with haloperidol and her psychotic symptoms improved. She was discharged and, for the first time, did not develop recurrence of the lesions over a 6-month period. She was then lost to follow-up.

There are two different types of factitious disorders: one that presents with psychological symptoms and another that presents with physical symptoms. The C-L psychiatrist usually encounters the physical type. This disorder is also known as *Munchausen's syndrome, pseudologica fantastica,* or *peregrination,* perhaps because patients with this disorder often have very elaborate histories and they get admitted into many different hospitals. There are several features in the clinical presentation that alert the C-L psychiatrist to the possibility of factitious disorder:

- Numerous surgical scars, usually in the abdomen ("railroad abdomen")
- Patient is evasive and argumentative
- Very colorful and dramatic personal and medical history
- History of multiple hospitalizations, malpractice, and insurance claims
- May be in the health care profession or related to someone in the health care profession

Symptoms in this disorder may be voluntarily produced in several ways:

1. *Total fabrications,* as in a 43-year-old woman who complains of severe abdominal pain and yet there is none.
2. *Exaggerations,* as in the 30-year-old man who has a mild headache and acts as if he has the worst imaginable headache, such that he wants to split his head.
3. *Simulations of the disease,* as in the 60-year-old man who pricks his finger and drops it into his urine so that he will show hematuria and be worked up.
4. *Self-induced disease,* as in the 55-year-old woman who injects her urine into her IV to cause sepsis.
5. *By proxy,* where there is an intentional production of feigned physical or psychogenic symptoms in another person who is under the individual's care (usually a child). The motivation is to experience the sick role or the caregiver role through another person.

There is an art to managing these types of patients. Quite often, once confronted, they become very incensed and leave against medical advice. It is also a problem when we label these patients as "factitious" because our colleagues in the medical profession will then stop trying to find a physical cause for the symptoms. This would then lead to failure to diagnose a serious physical disorder, which the patient may actually have.

In managing these patients, we need to first rule out the presence of comorbid psychiatric conditions and treat them if they exist. It is important to emphasize the explanation for the symptoms and arrange for regular brief follow-ups. We need to minimize polypharmacy and multiple costly diagnostic tests, unless truly indicated. It is necessary to carefully go over the medical history, particularly what tests have been done, and avoid repeating tests. Patients, even if they have factitious disorder, are entitled to at least one good medical workup. Finally, specific treatment should be provided when it is indicated. Remember that what appear to be factitious symptoms may mask the presence of a *bona fide* illness.

MALINGERING

Malingering is an intentional production of false or exaggerated symptoms motivated by external incentives such as obtaining compensation, drugs, avoiding work, military duty, evading criminal prosecution, or influencing the relationship with another person.

CASE VIGNETTE: "OLD-FASHIONED LIE"

A 40-year-old man was brought in to the medical ER by police who found him wandering aimlessly on a busy parkway. The patient reportedly did not know who he was and where he was. He claimed that all he could remember was walking around the parkway trying to find anything familiar to him. Workup for neurologic disorders did not reveal any abnormality. Psychiatry was called to see the patient. An interview with the patient revealed inconsistencies. After confronting the patient, he admitted he was running from drug dealers and that he thought the hospital was a safe haven from them.

Although this type of behavior can be seen in any diagnostic category, it is not viewed as a specific type of disorder. This is the intentional fabrication of symptoms to achieve a secondary gain, which is usually material benefits. It is quite common in psychiatric ERs in the winter, when homeless people claim to be suicidal and depressed to gain admission for "3 hots and a cot." In the C-L setting, we see patients who request for disability benefits and claim to be physically disabled when they are not or the motor vehicle accident victim who reports serious injuries when they are not really present. It is also common in the forensic population. Prisoners will ingest foreign bodies to get out of their tiers and be placed in the forensic psychiatric units. Often, the C-L psychiatrist will act as an investigator who tries to verify information in the course of evaluating the patient.

LIAISON POTENTIAL

1. Work closely with the medical staff when dealing with these patients.
2. Hold psychiatric clinics in ambulatory medical settings.
3. Educate clinicians in recognition of symptoms that suggest somatization.

14 ▼ Pain Management

Essential Concepts

- The most important tool in good pain management is an appropriate assessment. This assessment should be repeated and it should be systematic.
- Tolerance and physical dependence are pharmacologic properties of opioids and do not necessarily mean "addiction."
- Pain management should be individualized. There is no given dose of a drug that provides analgesia for all patients. Pain is subjective, and therefore we cannot presume to know how a patient should be feeling.
- There is no ceiling dose for opioids, but there is a ceiling dose for nonopioids, such as acetaminophen, aspirin, and nonsteroidal anti-inflammatory drugs (NSAIDs), above which the drugs can cause liver and kidney damage.
- The use of adjuvants, as well as nonpharmacologic interventions, may minimize the need to increase the doses of opioid analgesics and should always be considered when pain relief has not yet been obtained. They should be part of an integrated approach to good pain management.
- The bottom line in pain management is to answer these questions: Is there pain relief? Is the patient able to function? Are there side effects to the medications? Is the patient exhibiting aberrant drug taking behaviors?

Pain is one of the most common symptoms that is seen in the hospitalized patient. Unfortunately, it is also one of the most undertreated symptoms. Pain involves not just the perception of a sensation, but the emotional reaction to it as well. In 1979, the International Association for the Study of Pain defined pain as "An unpleasant sensory and emotional experience associated with actual or potential tissue damage, or described in terms of such damage. Pain is always subjective. Each individual learns the application of the word through experiences related to injury in early life." Clinically, this means that "pain is whatever the patient says he/she is feeling."

The inadequate management of pain affects all aspects of a patient's life. Therefore, it is not surprising that a psychiatrist often is involved in the overall management of a patient's pain. In many hospitals, particularly since the Joint Commission for Accreditation of Hospitals has focused on pain as a "fifth vital sign," there are pain management teams. Ideally, these teams should be multidisciplinary. Usually, they are limited to anesthesiologists and/or oncologists. As a consultation-liaison (C-L) psychiatrist, you will see patients who get referred for depression, suicidal ideation, behavioral problems, or "drug-seeking" behavior. Very often, after a complete evaluation, we recognize that the underlying problem is that of inadequate pain management. It is important, therefore, that you be knowledgeable in this area, even if there is a pain management team. While this chapter is not an all-inclusive primer in proper pain management, we attempt to provide a working knowledge on this important issue to assist you when you see these patients.

BARRIERS TO APPROPRIATE PAIN MANAGEMENT

The Fear of Addiction

Concerns about the risk of addiction play a significant role in limiting the use of opioid analgesics for those who need them. Addiction is not the same as physical dependence and tolerance. Physical dependence (the emergence of a withdrawal syndrome on abrupt decrease or discontinuation of a drug) and tolerance (the need for increasing doses to achieve the same effect) are pharmacologic properties of the medications. Addiction, on the other hand, is a behavioral syndrome that involves, among others, the compulsive use of a substance, preoccupation with that substance, continued use despite harm, and other aberrant drug-taking behavior (Table 14.1).

TABLE 14.1. Aberrant Drug-Taking Behavior

More predictive	Less predictive
Selling prescription drugs	Aggressive demand for more drug
Forging prescriptions	Drug hoarding
Stealing or "borrowing"	Unsanctioned dose escalation
Frequent prescription "loss"	Unapproved use of the drug
Injecting oral/topical preparations	Unkempt appearance
Obtaining drugs from nonmedical source	
Concomitant use of illicit drugs	

(From Portenoy R. Opioid treatment for chronic nonmalignant pain: A review of critical issues. *J Pain Manage.* 1996;11(4):203–217.)

It is not just physicians and nurses who fear addiction, but some patients and their families fear it as well. This is particularly true in patients who have a history of alcohol and substance abuse and have maintained their sobriety for years. They fear that taking these medications will negate all the years of sobriety that they have achieved. Families sometimes also refuse pain medications for their child, spouse, or parent because of their fear of addiction. It is important to educate them to the fact that studies have shown that very few of the patients being treated in the medical/surgical setting who have legitimate pain actually develop an addiction. It is also essential to note that the opioid should be gradually reduced once the need for pain control no longer exists. Ideally, this should be done while the patient is in the hospital, but, frequently, the patient is discharged before the time that this tapering is completed. If this is the case, a sufficient tapering dosage of the opioid should be given as an outpatient, until the tapering process is completed. Although you may not actually be the person who will prescribe this, you will need to make sure that the physician in charge of the patient does.

CASE VIGNETTE: INADVERTENT OPIOID WITHDRAWAL SYNDROME

A 43-year-old fireman suffered a 50% second-degree burn and had an extended 3-month hospitalization. He had required large dosages of narcotics, which effectively controlled his pain during the acute and healing phase of his wounds, and was in the process of being gradually tapered during the latter part of his hospitalization. He was followed up by a C-L psychiatrist during his hospitalization who helped him with his marked anxiety and depression, as well as his grieving for his losses and the adjustment to his new situation. The plan was to continue to see him as an outpatient after his discharge. On the evening of the second day after his discharge to his home, the patient beeped the psychiatrist. He reported that he was shaking with extreme anxiety and was in a cold sweat. He believed that he was having a panic attack. He could not stand this feeling and was quite desperate. He also was having fleeting suicidal thoughts. The psychiatrist determined that, on discharge, the patient who had not completed the tapering of his narcotic medication was only given a few extra strength acetaminophen (Tylenol) for pain. The patient was essentially pain-free, but appeared to be having an opioid withdrawal. The psychiatrist arranged for the patient to get some oral narcotic, which alleviated all his symptoms. The gradual tapering of the narcotic was then carried out over the next week, and the patient had no withdrawal symptoms at the conclusion of the treatment.

Inadequate Knowledge of Pain Management

Another common reason for undertreatment of pain is inadequate knowledge of pain management. In medical school and residency, not enough attention has been focused on pain management. Hopefully, this is changing now that the focus has been shifting. The lack of pain assessment skills is a deficiency among our health care providers. It is important that pain, a dynamic process, be constantly reassessed (Table 14.2). Repeated assessments, especially before and after treatments, are essential. There are several tools to assess pain. The most practical is the numerical rating scale in which the patient is asked to rate pain on a scale of 1 to 10. Proper documentation in the charts and titration of medication that is based on severity and etiology of the pain should be performed (Fig. 14.1). The lack of knowledge about the pharmacology of the drugs and current therapeutic approaches to pain management are very common reasons for poor pain control.

TABLE 14.2. ABCs of Pain Assessment

Ask about pain regularly and assess pain systematically
Believe what the patient is saying in his/her report of pain
Choose the appropriate pain control option
Deliver the interventions in a timely, logical, and coordinated
    manner
Empower the patient and his/her family to enable control of
    treatment to the greatest extent possible

(From Project Network, Memorial Sloan-Kettering Cancer Center, with permission.)

CASE VIGNETTE: IMPROPER CONVERSION

An obese 45-year-old woman had intra-abdominal surgery for a mass in the liver that resulted in multiple complications. The patient was on a ventilator postoperatively and was also receiving intravenous (IV) morphine (up to approximately 260 mg total per day for almost 2 weeks). She gradually improved enough to be sent to the regular unit. After a day in the regular unit, the patient started to become agitated. She was restless and quite belligerent and insisted on going home. The patient also was experiencing visual hallucinations. A stat psychiatric consultation was requested. Upon review of the patient's medications, it was noted that, on the first day of transfer from the surgical intensive care unit (ICU) to the

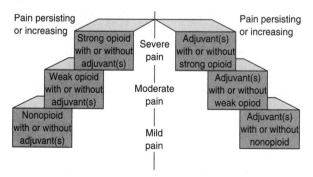

FIG. 14.1. Modified analgesic ladder. (From Project Network, Memorial Sloan-Kettering Cancer Center, with permission.)

regular floor, IV morphine was discontinued and the patient was placed on oxycodone and acetaminophen (Percocet) (two tablets every 4 hours, as needed, for pain). The C-L psychiatrist then recommended restarting the morphine in equianalgesic oral doses, after which a tapering schedule was started. The patient started to improve after morphine was given.

The above-mentioned case illustrates a common problem: the inadequate conversion from parenteral to oral doses or from one analgesic to another (Table 14.3). Another common mistake, as discussed in the preceding text, is using inadequate doses of medications. In some cases, the intervals between doses do not conform to the metabolism of the drug, such as giving the combination of 5 mg of oxycodone and 325 mg of acetaminophen (Percocet) every 8 hours when the medication effect will only last approximately 4 hours. Often patients are given drugs on an as-needed (p.r.n.) basis, rather than around the clock. By the time the patient actually gets his or her medication, the pain rating is much higher. If this is the case, you may need to be an advocate for the patient. In addition, the level of the medication is not consistently therapeutic if given on a p.r.n. basis. There are times when the levels are high, which causes more side effects or toxic effects, and times when the level is too low, which causes severe pain to recur. One important issue that many of our colleagues seem to forget is the importance of utilizing adjuvant drugs (e.g., anticonvulsants, antidepressants, and others) as well as non-pharmacologic modalities [e.g., acupuncture, biofeedback, hypnosis, transcutaneous electrical nerve stimulation (TENS), and cognitive–behavioral techniques]. In the overall management of a patient in pain, these can help reduce the dosage of opioid drugs that may be needed to relieve pain. As a C-L psychiatrist, you should be familiar with these various modalities.

Fear of respiratory depression and other possible side effects of the opioid analgesics also interfere with appropriate pain management. Studies have shown that respiratory depression, although it may be a side effect, is unusual. Patients also develop a tolerance to the sedative and cognitive effects of opioids. Constipation is the most common side effect of narcotic pain medications, making it necessary for patients to get stool softeners or laxatives along with their opioids. Early recognition and aggressive treatment of the side effects and concern for them should not deprive the patient of the appropriate pain medications they require (Table 14.4).

TABLE 14.3. Equianalgesic Conversions—Adult

A guide to using equianalgesic dose chart:
- Equianalgesia means approximately the same pain.
- This equianalgesic chart is a guideline. Doses and intervals between doses are titrated according to individual's response.
- The equianalgesic chart is helpful when switching from one drug to another or switching from one route of administration to another.
- The longer the patient has been receiving opioids, the more conservative the starting dose of a new opioid.

Drug	Parenteral (IM/IV)	Oral (PO)	Recommended starting doses (patients >50 kg)		Onset (min)	Peak (min)	Duration (hr)
			Oral	Parenteral			
Codeine [also in combination with ASA (aspirin, acetaminophen)]	120–130 mg (IM)	200 mg	60 mg q 3–4 hr	60 mg q 4 hr (IM)	10 (IV), 10–20 (IM), 30–60 (PO)	30–60 (IM), 60–90 (PO)	3–4 (IM, PO)
Fentanyl (Duragesic, Actiq)	0.1–0.2 mg (IM)	25 µg/hr (TD)	Not available	Not available	1–5 (IV), 7–15 (IM), 5 (OT), 12–16 hr (TD)	3–5 (IV, 10–20 (IM), 15 (OT), 24 hr (TD)	0.5–4 (IV, IM) 2–5 (OT), 48–72 (TD)

Continued

173

TABLE 14.3. Continued

Drug	Parenteral (IM/IV)	Oral (PO)	Recommended starting doses (patients >50 kg) Oral	Recommended starting doses (patients >50 kg) Parenteral	Onset (min)	Peak (min)	Duration (hr)
Hydrocodone (Vicodin also in Hycodan and Vicoprofen)	N/A	30 mg	10 mg q 3–4 hr	N/A	30–60 (PO)	60–90 (PO)	4–6 (PO)
Hydromorphone (Dilaudid)	1.5 mg	7.5 mg	6 mg q 3–4 hr	1.5 mg q 3–4 hr	5 (IV), 10–20 (IM), 15–30 (PO, PR)	10–20 (IV), 30–90 (IM, PO, PR)	3–4 (IV, IM, PO, PR)
Levorphanol (Levo-Dromoran)	2 mg	4 mg	4 mg q 6–8 hr	2 mg q 6–8 hr	10 (IV), 10–20 (IM), 30–60 (PO)	15–30 (IV), 60–90 (IM, PO)	4–6 (IV, IM, PO)
Meperidine (Demerol)	100 mg	300 mg	Not recommended	100 mg q 3 hr	5–10 (IV), 10–20 (IM), 30–60 (PO)	10–15 (IV), 15–30 (IM), 60–90 (PO)	2–4 (IV, IM, PO)

Methadone (Dolophine, Methadose)	10 mg	20 mg	20 mg q 6-8 hr	10 mg q 6-8 hr	10 (IV), 10-20 (IM), 30-60 (PO)	60-120 (IM, PO), 10 (SL)	4-8 (IV, IM, PO)
Morphine (MS Contin, MSIR Roxanol, Oramorph)	10 mg	30 mg ATC 60 mg single dosing	30 mg q 3-4 hr	10 mg q 3-4 hr	5-10 (IV), 10-20 (IM), 30-60 (PO, PR)	15-30 (IV), 30-0 (IM, 60-90 (PO, PR)	3-4 (IV, IM), 3-6 (PO), 4-5 (PR)
Oxycodone (Oxyir, Oxycontin, and Roxicodone; also in Percocet and Percodan)	N/A	20-30 mg	10 mg q 3-4 hr	Not available	30-60 (PO, PR)	60-90 (PO), 30-60) (PR)	3-4 (PO), 3-6 (PR)
Oxymorphone (Numorphan)	1 mg	10 mg (PR)	N/A	1 mg q 3-4 hr	5-10 (IV), 10-20 (IM), 15-30 (PR)	15-30 (IV), 30-90 (IM), 120 (PR)	3-4 (IV), 3-6 (IM, PR)
Propoxyphene (Darvon, Darvocet)	N/A	130 mg	N/A	Not available	30-60 (PO)	60-90 (PO)	4-6 (PO)

IM, intramuscular; IV, intravenous; PO, nothing by mouth; OT, transmucosal; NF, nonformulary; TD, transdermal; N/A, not available; PR, rectal; SL, sublingual; ATC, around the clock; SC, subcutaneous; SC = IM.

Courtesy of the Pain Committee, Westchester Medical Center, Valhalla, NY; McCaffery M, Pasero C, Pain: Clinical Manual, Mosby; 1999:241; AHCPR Guidelines — Acute Pain Management 1992, Drug Facts and Comparisons Jan 2000 8/00.

TABLE 14.4. Adverse Effects of Opioids

Constipation
Nausea/vomiting
Sedation
Changes in cognition, mood, and perception
Dry mouth
Pruritus
Urinary retention
Myoclonus
Respiratory depression

UNDERMEDICATION FOR PAIN

Staff-Related Factors

It must be recognized that many physicians and nurses, while they mean well and care a great deal about their patients, will undermedicate for pain. They convey the idea to patients that they should "hold out as long as they can before asking for the next pain medication." They will unwittingly contribute to the guilt complex that many patients develop for using narcotics during a hospitalization. Patients frequently feel that they are doing the right thing by trying not to ask for pain medication. (Some men might equate this with being "macho.") Often this is based on the shared erroneous belief among patients and staff that the patient is likely to become addicted to the pain medication. As noted earlier, this is not true. You can be quite helpful to patients by strongly encouraging them to ask for pain medication, as needed.

Physicians should be encouraged to write around-the-clock orders for pain medication rather than p.r.n., especially during the acute phase. Nurses need to be encouraged to give ordered medication (not to hold off or discourage the patient), as well as p.r.n. medication, unless there is a clear contraindication. When there are injuries to various limbs, movement and exercise of the affected limbs often will be encouraged early in the hospitalization to prevent contractures and to restore function. It is our observation that inadequate pain medication early in the hospitalization will discourage proper movement and lead to negative consequences. You can convey this information directly to patients, which may allow them to ask for and receive adequate pain control.

Patients who have been given long-acting paralytic agents, particularly in surgery or in the ICU, might have difficulty signaling that they are having pain. A similar situation occurs when patients cannot communicate because of being intubated. In the former situation, it might be possible for the patient to communicate "yes or no" responses by blinking his or her eye. In the latter situation, the patient may be able to write or point to words or numbers on a board. The C-L psychiatrist may be the person who establishes communication and conveys the fact that the patient's pain is not being controlled. Another way of determining that the patient may be in pain is to note the presence of agitation, restlessness, sweating, hyperventilation, tachycardia, and hypertension, all of which may be signs of anxiety that is accompanying pain.

The late Samuel Perry, a C-L psychiatrist at the Cornell Burn Center in New York, brought a psychodynamic perspective to the question of why patients are frequently undermedicated for pain. He suggested unconscious mechanisms that contributed to the staff's resistance to using more adequate dosages of analgesic. He felt that the patient's pain serves two important functions: it makes the patient a definable being, separate from the staff, and it helps to confirm that the "object" is alive. A pain-free disfigured burn patient might be experienced as "fading away" or in the "shadow of death." He suggested techniques that, as a C-L consultant, you could use to deal with these factors. You could point out differences between the caretaker and the patient. You also could help the staff see the patient as a well-defined separate individual by mentioning to the staff his or her struggles with various life events, such as adolescent children, recent purchase of a new home, worries over a failing grandmother, and so forth. It would also be helpful to describe to the staff some aspects of the patient other than the pain that makes him or her alive, such as his or her moods, fantasies, appetite, and the wish to be mobile.

Patient-Related Factors

It is not uncommon for some patients to underreport their pain for various other reasons. This can include the desire to please the staff and not be "a pain in the neck" for staff and the desire to have their doctor's focus more on the treatment of their primary problem. There are also cultural and personality factors that may influence the patient's presentation. For example, some patients appear stoic in the face of excruciating pain, whereas others can be hysterical after sustaining a very slight injury.

System-Related Factors

These factors include the fact that the availability of opioid analgesics is limited. Most pharmacies do not stock large amounts of opioids. In addition, specialized pain services are not available in every facility. Finally, pain management is not cheap, and some insurance plans may not cover the expenses of state-of-the art treatment. Therefore, insurance coverage versus out-of-pocket payments may not always be possible. As a C-L psychiatrist, you should advocate for good ethical care and should not accept this situation.

PSYCHOLOGICAL COMPONENTS OF PAIN

Patients who are in pain become quite anxious and are prone to feelings of dependency and helplessness. A severe injury often will bring out unconscious fears of dying, which can be related to deep-seated separation anxiety. There is a tendency for psychological regression under these circumstances. A depressed mood commonly becomes intertwined with anxious feelings. Sleep disturbances also occur.

Each of these factors heightens your patient's perception of pain, and any intervention that alleviates any of them can diminish your patient's suffering. Social interaction from family or friends is often very helpful. Indeed, we have noted that when family members visit patients in the hospital, the need for pain medication frequently diminishes. We also have found that if the patient believes that he or she has the support of the treating physician, nurse, or C-L consultant, he or she is likely to do better in regard to pain control. The patient needs to know that the staff is concerned and that they are doing everything they can do to relieve their pain and therefore much of their suffering. Various techniques, such as numbered pain scales, scales based on psychological factors, and visual analog scales, are used to communicate about pain. We believe that while these may be helpful in specific settings, nothing is better than an interested doctor or nurse who talks with the patient and cares about the pain that is being experienced by the patient.

PHARMACOLOGIC MANAGEMENT OF PAIN

Three major groups of pharmacologic agents that are used to manage pain are discussed briefly in subsequent text. Adequate pain management involves the use of one or more drugs from the different groups. It has been our experience that if combination drugs from different groups are used, there is less of a need to have higher doses of the opioids.

Nonopioid Analgesics

Aspirin and acetaminophen are common examples of the nonopioids, which also include all the different NSAIDs, as well as the newer cyclooxygenase-2 (COX-2) inhibitor drugs. These drugs are often used first line in the management of mild to moderate pain. There are many different NSAIDs with varying doses, and dosing should really be individualized. One of the more commonly used NSAIDs is ibuprofen, which is available in over-the-counter strength as well as prescription-strength doses. Aspirin, acetaminophen, and the NSAIDs are dose dependent and have ceiling effects. It is not uncommon that these drugs be overprescribed because of the reluctance of some physicians to prescribe opioids. However, you should be aware that high doses of acetaminophen can be toxic to the liver and, in some unfortunate cases, can cause liver failure and death. Chronic intake of high doses of NSAIDs, like ibuprofen, can cause renal failure. Gastrointestinal (GI) toxicity is also an adverse effect of aspirin (ASA), acetaminophen, and NSAIDS. COX-2 inhibitors, such as celecoxib and rofecoxib, are safer alternatives, but they can also be toxic to the kidney. It is part of your liaison work to educate those who are not as familiar with these toxic effects and are more concerned about the nonaddictive potential of these nonopioid drugs.

Opioid Analgesics

Opioids are generally classified as "weak" or "strong." They are available for administration through various routes: oral, parenteral, and transdermal. Most of the weak opioids are usually manufactured in combination with either aspirin or acetaminophen. Examples of these include acetaminophen and 60 mg codeine (Tylenol No. 4), oxycodone and acet-aminophen (Percocet), propoxyphene and acetaminophen (Darvocet), and so forth. There is a tendency for some physicians to overprescribe these combination drugs in lieu of prescribing stronger opioids. Unfortunately, they fail to realize that there is a ceiling dose for the NSAID and exceeding these levels causes more problems, without even achieving pain relief, than if they were to prescribe appropriate therapy. One other important caveat to remember is to identify side effects of opioids and to treat them aggressively.

Adjuvants

Adjuvants are medications that have other primary indications; however, they have been found to be useful in pain management. In fact, they have been used as single agents to manage specific types of pain. They include antidepressants, anticonvulsants, corticosteroids, alpha-adrenergic agonists, and others.

Antidepressants

Numerous studies have validated the efficacy of tricyclic antidepressants (TCAs) as a drug for the treatment of chronic pain. The most studied is amitriptyline, but others, such as imipramine, doxepin, clomipramine, and desipramine have been used as well. The selective serotonin reuptake inhibitors (SSRI)s have not been studied as well and studies thus far have yielded varied results. There have been favorable responses to paroxetine and citalopram, but more studies have to be done. You need to be careful about the anticholinergic side effects of the TCAs in particular, especially in patients who have cardiac problems, glaucoma, head injuries, and others. When used for pain, you usually need only low doses of the antidepressant and gradually titrate up to analgesic effect. TCAs have been shown to be particularly effective for neuropathic pain, especially with accompanying burning, numbness, or tingling sensations.

Anticonvulsants

Anticonvulsants have been used widely for neuropathic pain that is described as shooting, sharp, lancinating, or paroxysmal. The most commonly used anticonvulsant is gabapentin, and doses vary from 300 mg to as high as 3,600 mg. Other anticonvulsants, such as valproate, carbamazepine, phenytoin, clonazepam, and lamotrigine also have been used. When using these drugs, the side effects should be monitored. Newer anticonvulsants, such as topiramate and tiagabine, have not yet been used or studied extensively for pain management.

Miscellaneous Adjuvants

Although antidepressants and anticonvulsants are the most commonly used adjuvants, there are others that also are used. These include corticosteroids; alpha-adrenergic agonists, such as clonidine, mexiletine (an antiarrhythmic agent), and baclofen [a gamma-aminobutyric acid (GABA) agonist]; muscle relaxants; antihistamines; topical anesthetics, like capsaicin; and others.

Invasive Procedures

Usually considered after all other conservative options have been used and have failed, invasive procedures include intraspinal administration of opioids into the epidural or subarachnoid spaces. This approach allows the use of fewer opioids secondary to the amplification of the analgesic effect through this route. Other invasive procedures include temporary nerve blocks, trigger point injections, and neurolytic nerve blocks. Surgical interventions are sometimes used and include sympathectomy, rhizotomy, dorsal column stimulation, thalamic stimulation, and even frontal lobotomy. These have largely been supplanted by more conservative anesthetic techniques.

NONPHARMACOLOGIC MANAGEMENT OF PAIN

The appropriate management of pain involves treating the whole person. Pain affects all aspects of a patient's life and therefore it is necessary to utilize various techniques that do not just involve pharmacologic treatments. It has been long recognized that nonpharmacologic techniques significantly add to the analgesic effect of medications. It must be emphasized, however, that they are not usually effective when used alone. These include behavioral therapies, such as hypnosis and biofeedback, progressive muscle relaxation techniques, acupuncture, and cognitive behavioral techniques, such as distraction training, cognitive restructuring, and mental imagery, and physical therapy.

LIAISON POTENTIAL

1. Be a part of a multidisciplinary pain team.
2. Work with nursing staff and house staff to educate about the treatment of pain in a substance-abusing patient.
3. Start pain support groups in collaboration with the pain clinic.
4. Work closely with physicians treating patients with pain; see their patients daily.

Capacity Determination

> **Essential Concepts**
> - The term *competency* is a legal term ("*de jure*") and is determined by the judicial system, whereas *decisional capacity* is a clinical term ("*de facto*") that is used by clinicians.
> - Capacity determination changes as the nature of the patient's condition and the nature of the proposed treatment change.
> - Rational people can make what appear to be "irrational" decisions.
> - The psychiatrist's role is to assess for the presence or absence of psychiatric and/or cognitive impairments that interfere with the patient's ability to participate in decisions that are related to his or her care.
> - Informed consent is based on the patient's ability to understand his or her medical situation and participate in decisions related to that medical care.

You often will be asked by your medical–surgical colleagues to evaluate patients who refuse treatment or want to sign out against medical advice (AMA). This is especially true when the treatment team feels that the patient is not making a "rational" decision. For many, this means that the patient is not doing what the doctor wants him or her to do. Other common requests include the capacity evaluation of new mothers with psychiatric issues such as who will be taking care of their newborns or patients who refuse the discharge plans made for them

Oftentimes, we correctly assess that there is no impairment of the patient's capacity to make decisions, but that the problems lie in the communication between the patient and staff. It may be related to the struggle for control between them.

The liaison role of the consultation-liaison (C-L) psychiatrist is then highlighted. The determination of capacity is not exclusive to the C-L psychiatrist. Any attending physician can document whether or not a patient is capable of making decisions. Obviously, there would be no question about capacity in cases where a patient is comatose, severely retarded, and in a florid delirious or highly intoxicated state. It is when there is some question about the mental status that a formal psychiatric evaluation is needed.

In these situations, what we are about to evaluate is the patient's decisional capacity (*de facto* competency). This is different from legal competency (*de jure* competency), which is court determined, albeit based on the psychiatric evaluation. Determining capacity is usually fraught with vagueness, ambivalence, and many other psychosocial factors that exert a significant influence on the patient's decisional capacity. Once the patient is deemed capable of making decisions, he or she can make an informed consent.

INFORMED CONSENT

The doctrine of informed consent is central to the determination of the patient's capacity. If the patient has obtained the necessary information to make a rational decision, then he or she has the right to determine what can or cannot be done on his or her body. It is also incumbent upon the physician to inform the patient of all facts about his or her condition. Information that is given to the patient usually includes diagnosis, treatment, consequences, alternatives, and prognosis. If this is accurately provided to the patient and the patient voluntarily makes his or her decision, and if there is no psychiatric disorder that is interfering with his or her decision-making process, then the patient is capable of making decisions.

There are, of course, exceptions to this requirement for informed consent. These include the following: emergency situations that can mean the life or death of a patient, cases where there is an obvious lack of mental capacity or where the patient has been judged legally incompetent, cases where the patient waives his or her right to informed consent, and in cases of therapeutic waiver where the physician determines that informing the patient will cause more harm than good.

SHIFTING CAPACITY

Determining capacity is always specific to the case at hand at the particular time you are evaluating the patient. The questions that you ask focus around what specific decision the patient is making at that time. For this reason, it is important to ask the consultee what are they asking you to evaluate a patient's capacity for. This is necessary because a patient may be capable of making certain decisions and not others. Another reason is that a patient's capacity may shift during the course of the hospital stay. It can even change in the course of a few hours! On our C-L service, we often have seen patients early in the morning only to find a couple of hours later that the patient's mental status has taken a 180-degree turn!

DETERMINING CAPACITY

There is no universal law to follow when determining a patient's capacity. However, there are certain criteria that are widely accepted as guidelines. Experts have suggested similar criteria, which can be summarized as follows:

- Is the patient able to communicate a choice? Is the patient able to respond? Is there a thought disorder present? Does the patient have problems with memory? Is the patient able to explain his or her chosen decision? Is the patient ambivalent or is there vacillation?
- Is the patient able to understand the information presented? Is the patient able to repeat the information? Is the patient alert? Does the patient have deficits in attention span, intelligence, and memory? Does the patient understand the problem?
- Is the patient able to appreciate his or her situation and its consequences? Is the patient able to explain his or her illness and the need for treatment, as well as the outcome? Is there pathologic denial or are there delusions present that interfere with the perception of the situation?
- Is the patient able to reason and deliberate?
- Is the patient able to reach conclusions in a rational manner that are consistent with his or her own values? Is the patient psychotic, demented, delirious, depressed, extremely angry, or intoxicated?

On the basis of these criteria, we evaluate for the presence of any psychiatric disorder or mental condition that may interfere with any of the above. Remember that a patient can be schizophrenic and yet have the capacity to make certain medical decisions. The essential approach is to determine if the patient's mental illness (whether it is delirium, dementia, depression, schizophrenia, or other psychosis, etc.) is interfering with the patient's judgment for a particular situation.

We then focus on the nature of the decision the patient is to make. Decisions vary in significance, from having blood work done to having a transplant. Will a decision be a life or death one or will it hardly impact the patient at all? How much risk is there for the patient for how much benefit?

Drane recommended a "sliding scale" of medical situations to provide guidance for the capacity evaluation. You may also want to review websites mentioned in the appendix of this book

- For easy and effective treatments that are not dangerous and are for the patient's benefit, the requirement is minimal—only that the patient is aware of his or her medical condition and has given his or her consent.

CASE VIGNETTE: NO CAPACITY, BUT SURGERY PERFORMED

A 57-year-old male alcoholic was admitted after he fell and sustained a subdural hemorrhage. He was confused and unable to hold a conversation for a prolonged period of time. Shortly before his admission, he knew he had fallen and had asked to be brought to the emergency room (ER) to be treated. A capacity evaluation was done and he was judged unable to make decisions at the time. Surgery was done to evacuate the hematoma, without his written consent.

- For less certain treatments where the diagnosis is doubtful, the condition is chronic, or the treatment proposed is more dangerous and less effective, there are median requirements. The patient should be able to exhibit an understanding of his or her medical situation and the proposed treatment options and their risks and benefits. The patient makes a choice based on the outcomes.

CASE VIGNETTE: CAPACITY TO REFUSE TREATMENT

An 80-year-old woman with metastatic breast cancer was admitted for chemotherapy. She underwent a course of such therapy, but developed complications. She became dehydrated and unable to tolerate any oral intake. She refused to allow parenteral nutrition and had refused a second course of chemotherapy. We were called to evaluate her capacity to refuse treatment. Although her electrolytes were abnormal, the patient was sufficiently aware of her medical condition and was judged capable of refusing total parenteral nutrition (TPN) and another round of chemotherapy. She stated, "I have lived a good life. I tried to see if this will work. I don't think I want to live like this." She was subsequently discharged to be home with her family for the days she had left.

- For dangerous treatments, patients who make their own decisions must be able to appreciate the decision critically and reflectively. He or she must be able to demonstrate his or her ability to undergo a rational process to make the decision.

CASE VIGNETTE: PARENTS' RIGHT TO REFUSE LIFE-SAVING TREATMENT FOR 15-YEAR-OLD DAUGHTER

A 15-year-old female Jehovah's Witness was brought in to the ER after she was involved in a motor vehicle accident. She sustained multiple traumatic injuries and lost a lot of blood. She was unconscious, but her parents were able to come to the hospital almost as soon as she did. The physicians in the ER wanted to transfuse her with blood products, but her parents (acting in her stead) refused, despite the fact that they knew they could lose her if they did not transfuse her. The doctors refused to accept this and attempted to get a judge to override the family. Shortly thereafter, the uncle came with a living will where the patient had expressly stated that she did not want blood transfusions under any circumstance. The patient was then not given a transfusion and soon died.

As mentioned earlier, there is really no official consensus about the criteria for making capacity determinations. In most situations, the patient's consent or refusal is balanced with the risk–benefit ratio of the proposed treatment. When the patient consents to a treatment that has low risk and will be of high benefit to the patient, the test for capacity is low; however, if the patient refuses, then a higher test for capacity will be needed. Each case is different and, for each individual patient, the decision applies to the situation at a certain point in time (that is the time of the evaluation). Every patient needs to be reevaluated as his or her situation changes. If there is a conflict, then the issue needs to be brought before a court who will make a determination of the patient's competency.

16 Psychodynamic Issues and Psychotherapy in the Consultation-Liaison Setting

---

Essential Concepts

- Grief work is an important type of therapy for most hospitalized patients.
- A patient's anger toward hospital staff often is displaced from anger and frustration toward oneself.
- Encourage your patients to express their secret fantasies about the meaning of their illness or injury.
- Time-limited psychotherapy is a useful technique in the medical/surgical setting.

Any interaction that you have with a patient in the medical/surgical setting has psychotherapeutic potential. The doctor–patient relationship is a powerful one and, in the hospital setting, it is often symbolic of the parent–child relationship. The patient is ill, vulnerable, and dependent, and wants to be taken care of. This can be seen in its most extreme form in the intensive care unit (ICU) where the patient is totally dependent on the medical staff, but there is always a spectrum of dependency. You will be asked to see patients who are in full control of their decision-making power and, in these cases, the patient–doctor interaction is between two mature adults discussing the best course of treatment for the patient. As a consultation-liaison (C-L) psychiatrist, you will have the opportunity to evaluate and help improve the relationship between doctor and patient.

CASE VIGNETTE: MODELING DOCTOR–PATIENT RELATIONSHIP

A 38-year-old man with severe infection requires continued intravenous (IV) treatment for a 2-week period. The treating internist is very attentive to the care of the patient and makes numerous visits to adjust the medication and examine the patient, but does not explain to the patient the reason for the treatment and any possible options for outpatient treatment. The patient does not ask any questions, but tells the staff that he is very unhappy and wants to sign out, against medical advice. When the nurses inform the physician of this intent, he calls up the patient's significant other and explains how it is essential for continued IV treatment. Finally, the C-L psychiatrist is called into the picture and arranges a joint meeting with treating physician and patient. The contrast of the psychiatrist addressing the patient with respect and interest in his concerns and wishes becomes obvious, and the treating physician begins to enter into dialog with the patient. This leads to an adult–adult interaction, with the beginning of a trusting relationship on a mature level, between the two of them.

There are many psychotherapeutic techniques available for your work with medical and surgical patients. In this chapter, we describe some of these and offer suggestions for which techniques might be appropriate for particular situations.

CATHARSIS OR VENTILATION METHOD

Patients who are ill enough to be hospitalized are (suffering) usually in both physical and emotional distress. While this may go without saying, it is ironic how little opportunity there is for patients to discuss the details of their illness or injury in an open-ended manner. This is where you come in. Before asking a lot of diagnostic questions, allow the patient ample time to talk about his or her illness and to express associated fears, uncertainties, sadness, and grief. This expression of feeling, known technically as *catharsis* or *ventilation*, can be quite therapeutic in and of itself, even in the absence of fancy interpretations and other psychotherapeutic techniques.

GRIEF WORK

Physical illness or injury usually brings with it some kind of serious loss or threatened loss. Your patient may not be able to function in his or her former roles as worker, parent, or spouse as he or she did before. The loss may be dramatic, such as in the case of a stroke or major surgery, or the loss may be more gradual, as with a slow-growing cancer or other chronic illness. Many people have a secret fantasy of immortality and serious illness punctures that fantasy. Be sure to spend time with your patient in understanding the deeper meaning of his or her loss. Often things are not what they seem.

CASE VIGNETTE: THINGS ARE NOT WHAT THEY SEEM

A 26-year-old artist experienced a traumatic amputation of her dominant arm in an automobile accident. By the end of the first week of hospitalization, the medical and nursing staff voiced concern that the woman had expressed no sadness about being unable to paint. During a C-L consultation, the patient stated that she really had wanted to pursue another career and could handle the fact that she would not paint again; however, she was devastated by the thought that she would never be able to embrace fully the baby that she dreamed of having one day.

Grief work is a term that is applied to the process of mourning and the intrapsychic readjustment necessary for the resolution of loss. In her work on death and dying, Kubler-Ross discussed five states of grief: denial, bargaining, anger, depression, and acceptance. In the medically ill patient, issues involved with grieving include loss of health, loss of function, and loss of the fantasy that he or she will have a "longer life" than is realistic. Not every person goes through all stages, and the stages may not be in a particular order.

In your therapeutic interactions with patients who are undergoing loss, you can facilitate the necessary grief work by using some the following approaches:

Acknowledge the loss—As a mental health professional, you are allowed (and even expected) to bring up subjects that family and others avoid. Once the loss is out in the open, the patient often is willing now to talk about it. Empathic statements such as, "This must have been a very painful loss for you" often promote an outpouring of emotion.

Allow the patient to be with pain—Resist the temptation to divert your patient's thoughts from his or her painful feelings. Although it may feel natural to try to point out "positive" aspects of the loss to comfort your patient, far more helpful words to the grieving person are, "I can see you are in a great deal of pain. Tell me more about what that feels like." Such encouraging words as, "A time will gradually come when the pain will not be so intense or so ever present" are appropriate, after the patient has done some initial grief work.

Normalize your patient's pain—Patients may feel they are losing their minds because of the intensity of their distress. This can be a time to reassure them that these are common feelings and will pass over time.

Provide assurance by exploring past coping patterns— Ask your patient to describe the most difficult thing he or she has ever endured in the past and how he or she managed to endure it. This can be reassuring, as it gives the patient more courage to deal with his or her current devastation. Beware that in this process, the pain of previous losses that have not been experienced fully may be rekindled.

Monitor danger signals during grief work—While diminished appetite and sleep are common during grief and do not necessarily indicate a major depression, if they are severe or persist for several months, pharmacologic treatment for depression may be required. Fleeting thoughts about giving up are not unusual, but any active suicidal ideation must be explored and monitored carefully. We have found that grieving persons may try to increase their use of tranquilizers, antidepressants, or pain medication in an attempt to self-medicate and numb themselves from the pain of grief.

Family—Be alert to the possibility that your patient's family may not understand the grieving process that is being played out. If necessary, do some psychoeducation about the normalcy of loss, grief, and mourning. Be aware that family members may themselves be grieving.

PSYCHOTHERAPEUTIC APPROACH TO ANGER

Patients in the medical setting are frequently angry. Your patient may be angry at the simple fact of being hospital bound. At other times, your patient may be angry at the hospital or medical staff for reasons such as delays on receiving medication or in responding to calls, transportation errors, perceived rough handling, visits by medical staff that are considered to be too brief, poor communication by staff, and so forth. Expressions of anger are usually muted because patients have a natural reluctance to criticize the medical and nursing staff on whom they are so dependent. A simple inquiry often allows a patient to express emotions that were boiling close to the surface. An empathic statement such as, "I understand how, at times, you get very angry and frustrated," can be comforting and supportive. There is usually no need to redirect the anger or attempt to talk the patient out of any such feelings. Family members and friends, on the other hand, are often uncomfortable with these emotions and they may try to divert the patient from them. Therefore, your meetings with the patient take on an added importance, giving your patient the sense of a "safe place" to express anger.

At times, the patient's anger gets out of control. In such situations, family members who are objects of this anger can be brutally antagonized. Old conflicts are rekindled without any apparent reason. The patient also may express hostility toward the medical and nursing staff. He or she may refuse medications and procedures or threaten to sign out against medical advice. Noncompliance is one of the few acting-out behaviors available to the hospitalized patient.

When asked to consult in such situations, your first course of action should be to clarify and correct any simple problem (although problems are rarely simple). Encourage your patient to ventilate and express his or her feelings. You may want to prescribe a brief course of benzodiazepines, if the situation is acute.

CASE VIGNETTE: THREE EXAMPLES OF DISPLACED ANGER

Example 1: A 56-year-old man who was 48 hours post open heart surgery was taken to radiology for a chest x-ray. The patient claimed that his doctor did not tell him about the study. His attentive family encouraged him to go for the x-ray and not to ask so many questions. Just before the x-ray was to be taken, it was determined that this was the wrong patient and indeed he was not scheduled for a chest x-ray. The patient was returned to his room where his meal was cold. He became very angry and refused to eat his food or take his medications. A psychiatric consultation was called and the nature of the patient's anger was quite clear. He was angry with the staff for the mistake that they had made, with his family for discouraging him from complaining, and at himself for not speaking up. It was also easy to help him acknowledge that people in the hospital are often afraid to speak up because they are afraid that they might offend the caregivers on whom they are dependent upon for care. The nature of this feeling and his right to speak up was discussed, as was the understanding that a more serious mistake could have been made. This discussion was quite therapeutic for the patient.

Example 2: A 48-year-old woman had a recent diagnosis of recurrent ovarian cancer and was having a diagnostic workup in the hospital. Her older sister visited her regularly in the hospital. At a time of inclement weather, the sister missed a visit. During her next visit, the patient expressed tremendous anger at her sister's absence the previous day and called it "the typical way the sister always treated her as a child." The patient also concluded that she was wasting her time in the hospital because "doctors were taking their time and doing too many tests." She then expressed her intention to sign out, against medical advice.

Example 3: A 26-year-old patient was being treated in the burn unit for electrical burns in his hand that he sustained in his work as an electrician. He required an abdominal flap to graft skin from his abdomen to his hand. After 3 weeks in an uncomfortable position, the graft failed and the procedure was scheduled to be repeated. The patient was angry and frustrated. He blamed the doctors and nurses in the unit for not caring for him properly. He wanted to leave the hospital and go to another facility, although he knew that his current hospital was well known to have outstanding expertise in this procedure.

In many other cases, we have found that the patient's anger is being displaced on external objects. Unlike earlier examples of patient anger that required only an empathic acknowledgment, a skillful therapeutic maneuver with a delicate interpretation is now in order.

INTERPRETATIVE ANGER AT SELF

To make the right kind of interpretation, you have to realize that these patients are, in reality, also angry with themselves.

They are angry about their own role, real or imagined, in their illness or accident. This may include a deep-seated anger at themselves for having been overweight, for smoking, for bad dietary habits, for having skipped medical checkups, for drinking at the time of the accident, and so forth. Patients may become angry with themselves for not recovering fast enough, for needing pain medications or not tolerating the testing, and for the hospital situation. They often have an anger and disappointment at their own body for failing them. These feelings are mostly unconscious and unacceptable and this is why they are displaced onto external objects such as staff and family.

In this situation, you must decide whether to interpret the true nature of the anger. A typical interpretative statement might be, "While you are blaming the doctors for not recovering fast enough (or at your family for not visiting, etc.), I think you are really mad at yourself for becoming sick (or for the accident you had, etc.)." Be aware that this technique can sometimes precipitate a severe depression, as patients become painfully aware of the anger directed toward themselves.

A more gentle approach is to suggest that the patient's anger is directed toward an intermediary object. For example, in attempting to diffuse displaced anger toward the medical staff, your interpretation might deal with anger at the "illness" or the "accident." This statement might be "While you are expressing all this anger at your family for missing visits or the doctor for doing so many tests, I think that you are really furious at the damn cancer that you are fighting." This indirect or "inexact" interpretation often allows the patient to redirect his or her anger away from the people who are trying to support them and put it close to the source of their psychological pain. Yet, by still keeping the object external (the "illness" or the "injury"), it minimizes the self-blame that can be so devastating.

There is always the possibility that you will become the object of the patient's anger, either by the same displacement mechanism or because the interpretation is experienced as "hurtful" in some way, perhaps because it is too close to the source of the pain. This possibility can be minimized by avoiding interpretations early in the consultation process before a positive relationship with the patient has been established. This positive relationship may happen at the tail end of an initial consultation after the patient has experienced your empathic and caring attitude. Or it may be necessary to wait until a follow-up visit to the patient. Sometimes, you may have little choice but to try to diffuse the anger early on, but, of course, you should be prepared to handle the angry feelings directed toward you.

CLARIFYING PATIENT FANTASY ABOUT ILLNESS OR ACCIDENT

Your patient usually has her own secret idea about the cause of the illness or injury. As part of your therapeutic work with a patient, explore this fantasy. We suggest some variant of the following approach: "You know, everyone usually has some secret thoughts about why they are sick (or why they had this trauma). Often these private ideas have nothing to do with the medical facts or apparent circumstances, but they are meaningful to the person. Can you share with me your thoughts about why you are in this condition?"

Frequently, patients will express guilty feelings, as if it were a punishment by God or some higher force or an act of fate against them. Some may fantasize that they are being punished for earlier deeds, such as for not having been a good child. Often the fantasy relates to the patient's psychodynamic personality structure. The dependent depressive patient, for example, may speak about a sense of inadequacy and a poor sense of self-worth.

The obsessive patient may not be able to make up his or her mind concerning the fantasy. A patient who thinks concretely might find it difficult to have any fantasies whatsoever. Such information is always useful in subsequent psychotherapeutic work with patients.

THERAPEUTIC VALUE OF "BRUSH WITH DEATH"

Any serious illness, injury, or, in fact, any condition that leads to a hospitalization will remind most people of their own mortality. Time spent in the ICU is almost always experienced as "a brush with death," and the usual psychological defenses against facing death are lowered. This can cause intense anxiety. It also causes a regression to more vulnerable child-like feelings and the wish to be cared for by parental figures and parental substitutes.

There is also a tendency to "take stock." When the sense of immortality is taken away, there is an opportunity and motivation for an honest self-assessment. This is similar to a "midlife crisis." In such a crisis, a person believes that he or she has a last chance to make important changes in life. He or she can be mobilized to act and make changes in the marital relationship or to take such actions as buying a coveted sports car or desired jewelry or choosing a new career. A hospitalized trauma patient who is integrating a brush with death also may go through this midlife crisis. This occurs regardless of the person's age. The patient may begin to plan changes for the future and is often receptive to positive psychotherapeutic interventions. Patients may now be more willing to make serious lifestyle changes in regard to exercise, eating habits, or alcohol or drug use.

Asking your patient "How has your illness or accident changed your life?" can be a good entry into his or her thought process on this topic. Picking up on statements, such as "I better change my life before it is too late," can lead to further clarification and may lead to a referral for psychotherapy.

PSYCHODYNAMIC LIFE NARRATIVE TREATMENT APPROACH

Viedermann and Perry have suggested an insight-oriented psychotherapeutic technique to treat depression in the physically ill. The authors found that medically ill depressed patients show three important characteristics:

1. Psychic disequilibrium with confusion and uncertainty
2. Regression with intensified transference
3. A tendency to examine the trajectory of one's life—where one has been, where one is going, and which expectations will be fulfilled

Viedermann and Perry described their suggested interventions as a "psychodynamic life narrative" because it is a global statement about the meaning of the illness or injury in the context of the patient' entire life, as opposed to the interpretation of a single conflict. Using this approach, the first step is for the therapist to examine the patient's present and past life, with emphasis on psychological factors and relationships. This can usually be done in two or three bedside consultation visits. During these contacts, the information gathered will be used ultimately in formulating the psychodynamic life narrative. In these preliminary visits, the therapist may be making clarifying statements, empathic statements, or perhaps recommendations to the medical staff concerning psychotropic medications or pain control.

At some point, the therapist will have enough information to make a "psychodynamic life narrative interpretation" to the patient. This statement explains what the illness or injury means psychodynamically to the patient at this particular time. The degree of depression is framed as a natural result of the patient's personal psychology, rather than as an inevitable consequence of the illness itself. The narrative is designed to create a new perspective and to increase self-esteem through the emphasis of past strength, supports, and coping mechanisms that the patient has found to be effective. The interpretation will be better received if it is presented in an engaging and vigorous manner that conveys fascination and interest in the patient, as well as affirmation and hope.

CASE VIGNETTE: THREE EXAMPLES OF THE USE OF PSYCHODYNAMIC LIFE NARRATIVE INTERPRETATION

Example 1: A 59-year-old woman with cancer of the breast had to undergo a radical mastectomy, which needed to be followed by radiation and chemotherapy. The prognosis was considered quite good and her husband and large family were quite attentive to her. However, the patient became increasingly depressed. In preliminary consultation visits with her, she elaborated on how self-conscious she was that she was the only one among her five sisters who did not go to college, as most had advanced degrees, as did her husband and all her children. Yet, she was the glue that held the family together. She organized all family events and was very active in caring for infant grandchildren and in helping and solving other family crises. The narrative interpretation reviewed the role that the patient played in her family and how difficult it was for her to allow herself to be assisted and shepherded around by the family during the preliminary workup and evaluation of her cancer. The idea that she was too weak and tired to care for everyone was terrifying to her. She felt that this made her worthless and of no value to the family. The therapist reflected how it was interesting how her life trajectory and self-image were that she was only valuable by doing things for her family, when, in reality, even in her hospital bed, she was truly valued for the advice and love that she dispensed all the time. In fact, the therapist observed the friendly competition among family about who could spend time with her. This review and reforming of her feelings appeared to help her resolve her acute depression.

Example 2: A 31-year-old woman required a prolonged hospitalization with a good prognosis. She had numerous IV lines and was confined to a special mechanized bed, which made a constant humming sound as it rotated from side to side. She tolerated the sensory isolation of this procedure unusually well by making up stories to herself, but became depressed and tearful when she was moved into a regular bed and the IV lines came out.

During preliminary psychiatric interview, a history emerged of her being the youngest of several children and feeling neglected while growing up. She entertained herself as a child by making up imaginary stories. Later on, in high school and college, she was told that she was a talented writer. After graduation, she chose to work in her father's lumberyard, in an attempt to gain his approval. She had been thinking about going back to school to become a teacher or writer, but could not bear to tell her father about this plan. She was now concerned that she would not be able to do the physical labor required for her job in the lumberyard because of her illness.

In the psychodynamic narrative statement she was told, "You are now depressed because you believe that by not being able to work in the lumberyard you will disappoint your father and won't be a worthwhile person. Yet, you know that you want to be a writer or a teacher and are better than most in these endeavors. The reality is that this illness means that you won't be able to be as physically active as before, but that you can do what you always wanted to do."

When the patient responded to the life narrative, she acknowledged that she had felt neglected as a child. To make up for this situation, she suppressed her talents and wish to be a writer or to teach others to write. She was trying to please her father by working in his business, which her brothers had refused to do. The impact of this insight on the patient was quite dramatic. Her affect changed rapidly and she became quite receptive to the support of her family. She also began to reflect about the future in a more positive and realistic way.

Example 3: A 17-year-old Chinese–American male high school student was hospitalized with 28% second- and third-degree burns over his face and upper body. The injury occurred while he was repairing his parents' basement furnace. The patient was refusing to participate in physical therapy and was developing debilitating contractions. He was depressed and appeared to have given up and to have withdrawn into himself.

During a series of preliminary interviews that explored his background, the patient indicated that he did not think that he deserved to recover. Ultimately, a psychodynamic life narrative was made that pointed out how he had always tried to be a good kid—plodding away at school, working part-time, and never arguing with anyone, including his friends and family. He was told by the therapist that it appeared that he never got angry or lost his temper. "Of course, then, anger had to come out somewhere to keep you from exploding. It did come out in your dream that you had before the accident (a dream where the patient dreamed that he had blown up his house). Now, even though they found a defect in the welding equipment that caused the fire, you are convinced that your dream had come true and that you were trying to blow up your house. Because you have always been so good, you are now being extra hard on yourself for those angry feelings."

After the patient's suppressed anger had been placed in the context of his life and viewed as understandable adolescent rebelliousness, his depression began to lift and a therapeutic alliance was established for further work with the therapist.

TIME-LIMITED PSYCHOTHERAPY

We have found that a variation of the time-limited psychotherapeutic techniques of James Mann has been quite useful for the medical–surgical setting. Patients appropriate for such treatment might be patients who require extended IV therapy, such as those with oseteomyelitis or other infectious diseases; patients in traction, rehabilitation, or physiotherapy; and patients with persistent illness that requires extended or regular returns to the hospital, such as those undergoing transplants, cancer, or end-stage renal disease.

In your initial interview, try to identify a central conflict that is causing the anxiety or depression. In our experience, such conflicts often are reflected in interpersonal difficulties that exist before the injury. Problems with authority figures, dependency relationships, and separation issues are common examples. The presence of psychosis or profound depression is usually contraindicated in this technique. The patient should have a clear sensorium and be free of significant pain. Because this short-term psychotherapy approach usually involves a planned breaking off of contact with the psychotherapist at the conclusion of treatment, it might be advisable to have alternate referral sources for patients who are expected to have long-term severe psychological repercussions due to illness or injury.

With this technique, it is essential that the number of sessions planned, and their duration, be spelled out in advance. The usual technique described by Mann is 12 sessions of 45 minutes each, once per week. We have found it practical and workable to reduce the total number to six to eight sessions and usually to reduce the time to 20 to 30 minutes per session. The exact time of each appointment, including the final date, should be clearly specified in advance. This is based on the idea that knowing the termination date at the start intensifies the defenses against separation and loss and therefore serves to highlight the central conflict that will be dealt with in this therapy.

In the initial treatment sessions, allow your patient to ventilate, express feelings, and verbalize current concerns and conflicts. As the therapy moves into the second and third sessions, pay particular attention to any verbalizations that indicate positive transference, as well as any mention of the patient's awareness of the time-limited nature of this therapy. We recommend that you start each session by noting, for example, that "this is session number 4 of our planned eight meetings" and so forth.

This treatment technique is believed to be effective because the intense time-limited treatment technique mobilizes positive transference. In fact, there is often rapid symptomatic improvement within the first three or four meetings.

During the last couple of sessions, your patient typically will express emotions that are related to the impending termination of therapy. Sadness, grief, anger, and guilt are common, as your patient is not only dealing with separation from you, but also separation from the medical and surgical teams that provided care when he or she was helpless and frightened. An essential part of such psychotherapy is to examine feelings of termination as they relate to the present and the past. This will unavoidably become intertwined with the central conflict that had been the focus of the treatment.

As the therapist, you also may experience your own feelings of separation as termination approaches. Your awareness of such countertransference feelings can be helpful in understanding how other medical and nursing staff respond to this patient. At discharge, the entire treatment team may go through a separation process.

RELAXATION/MEDITATION TECHNIQUES

Many patients find that relaxation and meditation help alleviate even pain. Of particular note is the relaxation response, which has been described by Benson, that has been shown to quiet the body's response to stress. Research on these techniques has documented an immediate lowering of blood pressure, heart rate, breathing rate, and oxygen consumption. While there are many variations and sophisticated elaborations of this technique, there are two components that are the essence of this approach:

1. Focusing one's mind on a repetitive phrase, word, breath, or action
2. Adopting a passive attitude toward the thoughts that go through one's head

In regard to the focus on breathing, the relaxation technique usually works better when the patient can learn to do abdominal or diaphragmatic breathing rather than chest breathing. If the patient lies on his or her back and places the hands just below the belly button, the abdomen should be noted to rise and fall with each breath. This process can be facilitated by asking the patient to imagine a balloon inside of his or her abdomen. Each time the patient breathes in, he or she imagines that the balloon fills with air and, each time the patient breathes out, he or she imagines the balloon collapsing.

Simple instructions for the relaxation technique (with either just observing the breath or using a mantra) are listed in the subsequent text.

Observing the Breath

Sit in a comfortable position with your back straight and your eyes lightly closed, having loosened any tight clothing. Focus your attention on your breath without trying to influence it in any way. Follow the contours of the breathing cycle through inhalation and exhalation, noting the points at which one phase changes into the other. Do this for at least a few minutes. Your goal is simply to keep your attention on the breath cycle and observe it. No matter how the breath changes, just continue to follow it.

Using a Mantra

A mantra is a meaningful word or phrase that you repeat either silently or out loud during this meditation/relaxation technique. You can choose a holy name or brief prayer from your religious tradition or you can choose a neutral word or phrase such as "one," "peace," or "let go." As with the breathing exercise, assume a comfortable position and gently close your eyes. Take a few deep breaths. Then, let your breath come naturally and begin to repeat your mantra at whatever rhythm feels comfortable to you. If your mind begins to wander, gently bring it back to your mantra. Try this for at least a few minutes.

SUGGESTED READINGS

Benson H, Beary JF, Carol MP. The relaxation response. *Psychiatry* 1974;37(1):37–46.

Blumenfield M. Patients fantasies about physical illness. *Psychother Psychosom* 1983;39:171–179.

Blumenfield M, Schoeps M. *Psychological care of the burn and trauma patient.* Baltimore: Williams & Wilkins, 1993.

Jacobson E. *Progressive relaxation.* Chicago: University of Chicago Press, 1974.

Kubler-Ross E. *Death: the final stage of growth.* New York: Macmillan, 1975.

Mann J. *Time-limited psychotherapy.* Cambridge: Harvard University Press, 1973.

Vierderman M, Perry SW. Use of psychodynamic life narrative in the treatment of depression in the physically ill. *Gen Hosp Psychiatr* 1980;3:177–185.

Westberg GE. *Good grief—a constructive approach to the problem of loss.* Philadelphia: Fortress Press, 1962.

Substance Abuse Issues in the Medical Setting

because most hospitals are nonsmoking. Liaison work between the patients in nicotine withdrawal and the staff may help prevent acting out behavior [e.g., signing out against medical advice (AMA) because the patient cannot smoke].

Substance-abusing patients usually present to the hospital with a variety of physical complaints rather than with concerns about substance use itself. Making sure that a urine toxicology screen is done as soon as a patient presents will go a long way to help determine the presence of substance abuse and prevent the guessing game that usually follows when you suspect substance use but the patient vehemently denies it (Table 17.1). As a consultation-liaison (C-L) psychiatrist, you also have the opportunity to encourage the hospitalized patient to stop the abuse at a time when he or she is more receptive because of being faced with the medical consequences of the substance abuse.

ALCOHOL

Alcohol is a significant problem in the hospital setting. It may come in the form of alcohol intoxication, withdrawal, dependence, hallucinosis, pathological intoxication and, most important, delirium tremens (DTs). It is not unusual for alcohol abusers to deny or minimize their alcohol use. There are some markers in the laboratory results that are very suggestive of the presence of chronic alcohol abuse, such as elevated gamma glutamyl transferase (GGT) and other liver enzymes, macrocytosis as revealed by increased mean corpuscular volume (MCV), hyperlipidemia, and hypercholesterolemia. Useful tools to use in the diagnosis include the CAGE questionnaire (Table 17.2) and the first four questions in the Alcohol Use Disorders Identification Test (AUDIT) which address how often one drinks, how many drinks on a typical day, how often one drinks six or more drinks, and how often in the last year the patient realized that he or she cannot stop drinking once started. It is not difficult to recognize an intoxicated alcoholic. The patient usually has alcohol on his

TABLE 17.1. Approximate Duration of Detection in Urine Toxicology

Amphetamine and metamphetamines	48 hr
Barbiturates	
Short acting	24 hr
Intermediate acting	48–72 hr
Long acting	2–3 wk
Benzodiazepines at therapeutic doses	3 d
Cannabinoids	
Moderate smokers	3 d
Daily smokers	10 d
Daily heavy smokers	3–4 wk
Cocaine	6–8 hr
Cocaine metabolites	2–4 d
Ethyl alcohol	7–12 hr
Methaqualone	7 d
Narcotics	
Codeine	48 hr
Heroin	36–72 hr
Hydrocodone	24 hr
Hydromorphone	48 hr
Methadone	3 d
Morphine	48–72 hr
Oxycodone	24 hr
Propoxyphene	6–48 hr
Phenylcyclidine	8 d

(Adapted with permission from Hyman S, ed. *Manual of psychiatric emergencies*. New York: Little, Brown and Company, 1988:334.)

TABLE 17.2. CAGE Questionnaire

C — Have you felt the need to Cut down on your drinking?
A — Have people Annoyed you by criticizing your drinking?
G — Have you ever felt bad or Guilty about your drinking?
E — Have you had a drink first thing in the morning to steady your nerves or to get rid of a hangover (an "Eye opener")?

A score of at least two positive items indicates the need for detailed assessment.
(Ewing J. Detecting alcoholism: the CAGE Questionnaire. *JAMA* 1984;252:1905–1907, with permission.)

or her breath and gait is ataxic, mood is labile, speech is slurred, and nystagmus is noted. The patient can be given a benzodiazepine, along with thiamine and folate, and allowed to sleep. You will encounter these patients in the emergency room (ER), and it is often best to have them "sleep it off" before a complete psychiatric evaluation is done.

In the hospital setting, alcohol withdrawal can range from a mild uncomplicated withdrawal, which requires no medications, to florid DTs, which may require intravenous (IV) drip of benzodiazepines, neuroleptics, and restraints in an intensive care unit (ICU) setting.

Alcohol withdrawal can occur approximately 6 to 8 hours after a fall in the blood alcohol level (BAL). Severe symptoms begin 24 hours after the fall in BAL and may peak between 36 and 48 hours after the fall. Seizures can occur approximately 6 to 48 hours after abstinence. Withdrawal symptoms include increased blood pressure and heart rate, tremulousness, increased irritability, hyperreflexia, diaphoresis, hallucinations, seizures, and DTs.

Approximately 5% to 6% of alcoholics have the most severe form of withdrawal called *DTs*. This condition has a 5% to 10% mortality rate. It usually occurs after 3 days of abstinence. Symptoms include disorientation, profound autonomic hyperarousal, severe confusion, visual hallucinations, incontinence, diaphoresis, fever, gross tremors, and mydriasis.

When managing alcohol withdrawal, you should not just depend on the various protocols that are available (Table 17.3). Treatment should be individualized, using the protocols only as a guide. There can be no substitute for seeing the patient daily and adjusting the benzodiazepine, depending on the patient's presentation. Using chlordiazepoxide (Librium) provides a smoother detoxification, but you must guard against causing too much sedation due to the accumulation of the drug. Aspiration in an oversedated patient who is being treated with a chlordiazepoxide protocol is a rare, but potentially fatal, complication. Because of this, you should not forget to make sure "hold parameters" are in place. Keep in mind that you are not with the patient at all times. Another important issue is that chlordiazepoxide is better taken orally. Intramuscular chlordiazepoxide has an erratic absorption and should not be used. In patients who cannot take oral preparations and in patients who have liver dysfunction, using lorazepam (Ativan) is recommended. In severe cases, you may need to use lorazepam drip, along

TABLE 17.3. Alcohol Detoxification Protocols

Librium protocol: start only if patient shows signs of alcohol withdrawal	Ativan protocol: for alcohol-dependent patients with liver disease
Librium 50 mg q6h × 4 doses	Ativan 2 mg q6h × 4 doses
Librium 25 mg q.i.d. × 8 doses	Ativan 1 mg q.i.d. × 8 doses
Librium 10 mg q.i.d. × 8 doses	Ativan 0.5 mg q.i.d. × 8 doses
Librium 25 mg q6h p.r.n. for signs of withdrawal	Ativan 1 mg q6h p.r.n. for signs of withdrawal
Hold parameters: sedation and blood pressure <90/60 or pulse rate <60	Hold parameters: sedation, blood pressure <90/60 or pulse rate <60
Individualize the program for specific patients, as needed	Individualize the program for specific patients, as needed

with low doses of antipsychotics, if the patient has psychotic features or is severely agitated.

CASE VIGNETTE: TWO EXAMPLES OF ALCOHOL WITHDRAWAL

Example 1: A 50-year-old man was in a one-car motor vehicle accident where he lost control of his vehicle and hit a tree. He was conscious and fully oriented when he arrived at the hospital. He denied drinking and his BAL did not show intoxication. He sustained a compound fracture of the tibia, which required immediate surgery and general anesthesia. One day after surgery, he had a mild delirium with some confusion and disorientation. Brain imaging of his head to rule out head injury showed no pathology. The delirium was attributed to the anesthesia or his postoperative pain medication (morphine). By postoperative day 3, the delirium had worsened. He had severe tremor, was disoriented in all three spheres, and was responding to auditory and visual hallucination. He reported seeing small ants on the ceiling. Although the patient had initially denied any alcohol problems, his liver function tests suggested liver pathology, and family members later acknowledged that he was a heavy drinker. The patient was treated with the Librium alcohol withdrawal protocol and, within

48 hours, his sensorium cleared and he no longer had any hallucinations.

Example 2: A 75-year-old woman was admitted to the medical service for congestive heart failure. Her family was out of town at the time. Within 2 days of admission, the patient became confused and was noted to be hypertensive. Cerebrovascular accident (CVA) was the probable diagnosis, although brain imaging did not confirm it and there were no localizing signs. The patient then became paranoid and had visual hallucinations of seeing the devil outside of her room. The medical team began to consider that the patient was having side effects from her medications or possibly a toxic response to a cleaning chemical because her neighbor had reported that she was cleaning her house the day before admission. The patient's mental status did not improve, despite the institution of neuroleptic medication directed toward her psychotic symptoms. When the family was finally reached, they wondered if this condition could be related to the family secret that this sweet elderly woman was an alcoholic. The patient was immediately treated with Librium protocol and she had complete recovery in 3 days.

Both of these cases are illustrative of the fact that alcohol withdrawal can easily be missed if it is not suspected in situations where there is not a clear history of alcoholism. On the other hand, you should not be wedded to the sole diagnosis of alcohol withdrawal and DTs, especially if the patient does not show considerable improvement on the standard Librium or Ativan protocol within 48 to 72 hours.

When the patient who is no longer in delirium or withdrawal wants to stop alcohol use, there are several possible options. We recommend referring most of these patients to a 12-step group (such as Alcoholics Anonymous). A number of medications can be used to prevent craving, including naltrexone, desipramine, or the selective serotonin reuptake inhibitors (SSRIs). Disulfiram (Antabuse) can be used in highly motivated patients; however, Antabuse should be avoided in patients who have severe liver dysfunction, peripheral neuropathies, pregnancy, renal failure, and cardiac disease. In most situations, these medications should not be started until the patient is enrolled in an alcohol rehabilitation program where he or she will be closely monitored.

NICOTINE

Virtually all hospitals prohibit smoking in the patient's room and most nicotine-dependent patients who come to the hospital are not prepared to stop smoking. This is often a cause of patient–staff conflicts and acting out behavior.

CASE VIGNETTE: THE ANGRY SMOKER

A psychiatric consultation was requested for a 35-year-old man who was throwing things in his room. The patient was on isolation for treatment of multidrug-resistant tuberculosis. He had been acting out because he was not allowed to smoke. The patient was smoking surreptitiously in his bathroom. When his behavior was discovered by the staff, the patient's cigarettes were confiscated. He became quite angry and stated that he has been smoking for 20 years and that there was "no way" he was going to stop. He refused the nicotine patch and left his room, without a mask, to go out and smoke outside the building, without letting anyone know. He was then placed on constant observation and consultation was requested. The patient was throwing chairs and other things in his room at the time the psychiatrist came to evaluate him. He calmed down long enough to talk to the psychiatrist. The patient had no prior psychiatric history. He was very angry at what he felt was a violation of his rights. The psychiatrist was able to get the patient and the staff to agree to a compromise. The patient was going to be allowed to go to an inner courtyard in the hospital at prescheduled times during the day with his 1:1 staff, but he had to wear a mask until he reached the courtyard. Soon after this compromise was reached, the patient no longer presented a management problem.

As suggested by the case history, your liaison intervention, when the patient acts out in the hospital, is very important. You also can use this hospitalization as a form of leverage to try to convince your patient to stop smoking. Use the Fagerstrom Nicotine Tolerance Test (Table 17.4) as a tool to determine the level of dependence, as well as nicotine patch dosing (Table 17.5). Nicotine gum is another nicotine replacement alternative. You also can start the patient on bupropion (150 mg daily for 3 days and then twice a day for 7 to 12 weeks) provided he or she has no seizure history. If

TABLE 17.4. Fagerstrom Nicotine Tolerance Test

How soon after you wake up do you smoke your first cigarette?
- ☐ Within 30 min (1)
- ☐ After 30 min (0)

Do you find it hard to refrain from smoking?
- ☐ Yes (1)
- ☐ No (0)

Which cigarette do you hate most to give up?
- ☐ The first one in the a.m. (1)
- ☐ Any other (0)

How many cigarettes a day do you smoke?
- ☐ 15 or less (0)
- ☐ 16–25 (1)
- ☐ 26 or more (2)

Do you smoke more frequently during the first hours after awakening than the rest of the day?
- ☐ Yes (1)
- ☐ No (0)

What is the tar content of your brand?
- ☐ Low (0)
- ☐ Medium (1)
- ☐ High (2)

Do you inhale?
- ☐ Never (0)
- ☐ Sometimes (1)
- ☐ Always (2)

Total score: 1–6: low to moderate nicotine dependence
7–11: high nicotine dependency

the patient has not been successful with nicotine replacement therapy and/or bupropion therapy or these options are contraindicated for the patient, you can try varenicline (Chantix). Initial reports showed that this drug has been successful but more recently, the Food and Drug Administration (FDA) and

TABLE 17.5. Nicotine Patch

21 mg/d × 4 wk (6 wk in very heavy smokers)
14 mg/d × 4 wk
7 mg/d × 2 wk
Light smokers (<10/d) — no need to place on patch

the maker of the drug acknowledge that new onset of depressed mood, suicidal ideation, and behavior and emotional changes can occur within days to weeks of starting varenicline. Varenicline can also cause drowsiness. Patients on this medication need to be monitored and observed closely.

OPIOIDS: HEROIN, METHADONE, AND OPIOID ANALGESICS

Intoxication with opioids is easily recognizable because it includes drowsiness, miosis, dysarthria, and constipation. An opioid overdose (with heroin; methadone; and pain medications such as oxycodone, meperidine, morphine, and others) can result in stupor or coma, respiratory depression, pulmonary edema, and death. Severe opioid intoxication may require the administration of naloxone, an opioid antagonist, (0.4 to 0.8 mg IV every 3 to 5 minutes) until the patient becomes more alert and his or her breathing is normal. Always rule out opioid intoxication in a patient who presents with coma, miosis, and needle marks on his or her extremities.

Opioid withdrawal is not as life threatening as opioid overdose. Symptoms of withdrawal can be divided into early, middle, and late stages. In the early stage, there is lacrimation, yawning, rhinorrhea, and sweating. Restless sleep, mydriasis, anorexia, gooseflesh, restlessness, irritability, and tremors occur in the middle stage. There is an increasing severity of the above symptoms in the late stage, as well as tachycardia, nausea, vomiting, diarrhea, abdominal cramps, hypertension, depression, muscle spasms, weakness, and bone weakness. Withdrawal symptoms typically start approximately 6 to 12 hours after stopping opioids, peak in 2 to 3 days, and clear up in 7 to 10 days.

When managing withdrawal, we recommend using clonidine (Table 17.6), unless contraindicated (cardiac dysrhythmia, mitral or aortic insufficiency, or treatment with another antihypertensive). Methadone also can be used. However, be aware that you cannot discharge a patient who is on a methadone detoxification schedule because in most states only certified methadone clinics can dispense methadone for outpatient detox purposes. Therefore, you should only use it if you know that the patient will be in the hospital for a prolonged period of time, or at least during the entire detoxification period. Start with 30 mg per day and add 5 to 10 mg per day, based on the signs and symptoms of withdrawal. You can then taper by 5 mg per day.

TABLE 17.6. Clonidine Protocol for Heroin Withdrawal

Clonidine 0.2 mg q8h × 3 doses
Clonidine 0.1 mg q8h × 3 doses
May be given in doses of 0.1–0.2 mg q2h in some cases
Can be used with benzodiazepine
Obtain blood pressure before each dose and hold if blood
pressure is <85/55. Obtain orthostatic vital signs after
  administration. To be altered dependent on the patient's
  medical condition.

One of the issues that you face often as a C-L psychiatrist is a patient with "drug-seeking behavior." This is encountered usually when a patient is in pain and is asking for opioid analgesics. When there is a history of substance abuse (even if it is not opioids), there is a hesitation on the part of the physician to prescribe pain medications. Therefore, most patients with substance use history are undertreated for pain. (Chapter 14 provides a more extensive discussion.) However, there is always the possibility that the patient is indeed "drug seeking," so a careful evaluation is always essential.

COCAINE AND OTHER STIMULANTS

Cocaine is a potent stimulant known in the streets by various names such as "coke," "snow," "crack," "blow crack," "white lady," and "uptown." It is most often smoked or inhaled and also is injected or swallowed in powder, pill, or rock form. The highest addictive potential is with smoking crack, the freebase form of cocaine.

With cocaine, there is an intense short-term high that is followed by depression ("crash"). Prolonged use can result in hallucinations and paranoia. Most users develop a significant psychological dependence that is based on the positive rewards of the initial use. Intoxication is manifested by irritability, anxiety, talkativeness, dilated pupils, and sniffling. Tactile hallucinations ("cocaine bugs") also can occur. In severe intoxication, delirium can result. In the C-L setting, the important thing to remember is that cocaine causes a number of significant medical complications, even at the usual street doses. There is a significant cardiovascular toxicity with cocaine and it has been responsible for the sudden deaths of cocaine users. In addition, there can be nasal passage damage, lung damage, and liver toxicity.

Metamphetamine is a stimulant known as "crank," "speed," "crystal meth," "ice," and "black beauties." There has been an increase in the use of these drugs and it is not unusual to find patients who abuse them in the C-L setting. Treatment of the agitation and the psychosis seen in stimulant intoxication includes the use of antipsychotics and benzodiazepines, particularly lorazepam.

BENZODIAZEPINES

Benzodiazepines are quite commonly abused. In the 1960s through the 1980s, benzodiazepines were very popular medications for insomnia. It is particularly important that you ask patients specifically about "sleeping pills" because some patients may not know that they are taking benzodiazepines, but they know they take sleeping pills. One other issue is that benzodiazepine addicts often get their pills from various health care providers. It is important to get the patient's consent to contact his or her health care providers to get a better picture of what the patient is taking. When patients present with mental status changes, benzodiazepine withdrawal should be considered, if the history suggests use of benzodiazepines before the hospitalization.

Benzodiazepine intoxication can present in a variety of ways such as lability of mood, euphoria, or disinhibition to lethargy, ataxia, dysarthria, and nystagmus. In some cases, there may be blackouts or amnesic episodes. If the levels are high enough to cause respiratory depression, you can use flumazenil slowly, up to a total dose of 3 to 5 mg to reverse the effect of benzodiazepine. You need to be aware that this could precipitate benzodiazepine withdrawal.

CASE VIGNETTE: WITHDRAWAL FROM
SLEEPING PILLS

A psychiatric consultation was called to evaluate a 68-year-old woman who had had an emergency appendectomy 3 days earlier. The immediate postoperative period was uneventful. Three days after the surgery, the patient, who had no prior psychiatric history, suddenly became quite agitated and confused. She was seeing cockroaches flying in her room and was tremulous. Upon evaluation, the patient was noted to be unable to attend. The psychiatrist talked to the patient's husband, who denied that his wife had any alcohol history. Upon further investigation, the husband revealed that his wife had been taking a sleeping pill every night for the last 20 years. The psychiatrist was able to determine that the patient had been using triazolam. The patient was placed on tapering doses of clonazepam and eventually improved.

For benzodiazepine withdrawal, it is important to prevent seizures from occurring. You can use the original benzodiazepine or clonazepam (a long-acting benzodiazepine) in tapering doses.

The short-acting benzodiazepines are actually more addictive than the longer-acting benzodiazepines. Often it is difficult to switch the type of benzodiazepine. Once a patient is used to taking a particular type, some patients are resistant to changing the alprazolam, diazepam, and lorazepam that they have been on for a long time. It is recommended, however, to convert these benzodiazepines to clonazepam, which allows for a smoother detoxification (Table 17.7).

CLUB DRUGS

There has been an increasing trend in the use of "club drugs," which often are used in the club scene, usually in all-night parties, known as *raves*. The club drugs include methyldioxy methylamphetamine (MDMA) ("Ecstasy," "X"), so-called the "grandfather of all club drugs," gamma hydrobutyric acid (GHB), Rohypnol (the date rape drug), and special K (ketamine).

MDMA or Ecstasy is a dangerous drug that interacts with medications that are metabolized in the P-450 system. Its users

TABLE 17.7. Benzodiazepine Conversion to Clonazepam

Dose of clonazepam = dose of the benzodiazepine ×
(conversion factor)
Alprazolam: 0.25 mg (0.5)
Chlordiazepoxide: 25 mg (0.005)
Clonazepam: 0.125 mg (1)
Diazepam: 5 mg (0.025)
Lorazepam: 1 mg (0.125)

claim that "insights" and better relationships with people are positive effects of the drug. It has been implicated in the deaths of patients on antiretrovirals in Europe. More significantly, MDMA causes damage to central serotonin axons in the brain, severe liver damage, and malignant hyperthermia.

GHB abuse is also increasing. This drug is abused for a variety of reasons, including to treat insomnia, fight depression and stress, improve athletic and sexual performance, build muscles, and to get high. GHB intoxication can present with abrupt changes between agitation and somnolence or coma. In some cases, the agitation can be so severe that some patients may end up in the ICU, intubated and ventilated. Treatment is similar to alcohol withdrawal, with benzodiazepines.

Special K or ketamine is an anesthetic that is snorted, smoked, or injected intramuscularly. It can lead to hallucinations and a dissociative state ("K-hole"). Overdose or intoxication can lead to amnesia, depression, hypertension, delirium, and even respiratory depression.

The club drug scene is complicated by the fact that all the drugs described in the preceding text are frequently laced with other harmful drugs such as phencyclidine (PCP), cocaine, and heroin, which makes them even more dangerous and unpredictable.

LIAISON POTENTIAL

1. Educate staff (nursing and house staff, in particular) by doing in-services on substance use disorders, particularly updating them on the latest street drugs.
2. Develop a relationship through regular meetings or periodic contact with alcohol and drug rehabilitation programs. This will allow you to know the type of patients with whom these programs work best. It also can facilitate making referrals to these programs.

Disaster Psychiatry

Essential Concepts

- In addition to people directly impacted by disaster, there are secondary victims who may also be traumatized. This group includes police and fire personnel, emergency medical technicians (EMTs), and health care professionals including mental health workers, as well as members of the media.
- The unavailability of medication, usually taken on a regular basis, after a disaster can exacerbate both medical and psychiatric conditions.
- Research has now substantiated that Critical Incident Stress Debriefing (CISD) does not prevent long-term negative outcome and may create psychological difficulties in some people.
- The current overall psychological approach after disaster is aimed at fostering resilience, while managing acute stress and is known as *psychological first aid*.
- The application of Cognitive Behavioral Therapy techniques may reduce long-term post-traumatic stress disorder (PTSD).
- In situations of chemical and biological accidents or terrorism, the differential diagnosis between anxiety, panic, and delirium due to toxic etiology will need to be understood.

Psychiatrists and other mental health professionals who work in the consultation-liaison (C-L) setting can expect to be called upon to respond to disasters and threats of disasters or terrorist attacks along with the other members of the medical community. It would be a mistake to step back and say that you have not had disaster training and leave this task to others who may not be as qualified as you. Those who work with trauma or burn patients may feel more comfortable with this task and may have participated in planning for multicasualty events. The fact is that working on an everyday basis with medical illness, trauma, death, delirium, grieving, families, and children at the most difficult of times all prepares you for responding to disaster.

Having said this, there also is a strong case for taking training in disaster psychiatry before disaster strikes. There are courses given at the annual meeting of the American (Psychological) Psychiatric Association (APA) as well as an increasing number of lectures, seminars, and other continuing medical education (CME) available in many settings on this subject. There are also many journal articles and some new excellent books available. The APA web site, www.psych.org, has useful information immediately available for a quick review. Look on the home page under resources especially at the Disaster Handbook, which can be easily downloaded. The district branches of the APA have disaster committees, which can be joined as well as called upon at the time of an event.

As you become involved in this area, also keep in mind that there are many victims of a disaster in addition to the primary victims and their families. The police and fire personnel and EMTs are often psychologically traumatized by their experiences in assisting in the aftermath of a disaster. Similarly, doctors, nurses, and other health care professionals including mental health workers are impacted by the trauma as they attempt to help the primary victims of a disaster. Even members of the media who report on disasters, interview victims, and survivors and view the effects of these events are often traumatized. These secondary victims frequently deny that they are impacted.

GENERAL PRINCIPLES

Every disaster situation is different. There may be no survivors or relatively few physical injuries but large numbers of grieving families, friends, and coworkers. There are often many homeless and displaced people. After immediate care of physical injuries, attention is always directed to providing food and shelter as well as attempting to reunite families. Assisting with these basic needs while providing support can allow mental health professionals to gain the trust and confidence of victims of disaster. This also puts them in a position to recognize acute psychological problems in these victims. People who cannot care for themselves because of disorientation due to concussion or head injury or because of a dissociative reaction need to be immediately recognized. Among the first priorities are trying to be sure that people have medications, which they take on a regular basis. Particularly important are cardiac medications, antiseizure medications, and other medications for important medical conditions as well as antianxiety medication with potential for serious withdrawal effects, antipsychotics, mood stabilizers, and antidepressants. Psychiatrists can make efforts to see that these latter medications are included in emergency stockpiles in advance of a disaster and can be extremely useful in the proper distribution of them at the time of a catastrophic event.

Until fairly recently, Critical Incident Stress Debriefing (CISD), a group model where facts, thoughts, reactions, and coping strategies were discussed under the guidance of a group leader or a facilitator, was used in many varied settings. However, research has substantiated that there is no evidence that CISD prevents long-term negative outcomes and some studies have shown a higher incidence of negative outcome from this technique. The current overall approach is aimed at fostering natural resiliency, managing acute stress, and hopefully preventing long-term emotional problems although the research is still not clear how to successfully achieve this latter goal. The type of interventions recommended is being called *psychological first aid*.

PSYCHOLOGICAL FIRST AID

As described earlier, mobilizing support for basic needs (food, shelter, and medication), being sure that there are adequate living conditions, reuniting people with family members, and providing other social supports are essential. Families should be kept together whenever possible and there should be information available about the disaster situation and resources available. This can be done through in-person meetings, distribution of written material, mass media reporting, and through the Internet. Mental health professionals should be part of the team that prepares this material. Keep in mind that physical needs, interpersonal contact, and even educational information needed may vary from person to person and across cultural, gender, and social groups. You should try to be informed about cultural norms through community cultural leaders who understand the people who are affected. This may be particularly important when confronting rituals that have to do with death.

INTERACTION WITH DISASTER SURVIVORS

A good clinician who has worked in the C-L setting with physically ill, injured patients, and their families will have the experience in how to approach a person in the postdisaster situation in a nonintrusive, compassionate manner. This person needs physical and emotional comfort and needs to be listened to in regard to their immediate concerns. Providing warmth, nourishment, information, and other practical assistance will usually be the first step in the interaction. It may be necessary to calm and orient the overwhelmed survivor and sometimes, but certainly not always, a tranquilizer may be useful. All the proper precautions and anticipation of side effects should be taken into account when medication is administered. As noted, it is not necessary that the patient be encouraged to discuss or relive the recent emotional experience and, in fact, this could interfere with the natural recovery process. However, if the person wishes to do so, the clinician should be prepared to hear him or her out and, if appropriate, provide reassurance that the emotional response is understandable.

It can be useful to provide information and education about stress reactions and coping that will help the survivor deal with the disaster event and its aftermath. Every effort should be made to provide the person with information about available services that may be needed in the future. Ideally, this should be given in written form so it can be referred to later on.

PSYCHOTHERAPY

The environment is usually not conducive to doing formal psychotherapy in the immediate aftermath of disaster. Individual supportive sessions may be helpful and certainly individuals may resume previous psychotherapy, which will now deal with the recent traumatic event. Cognitive behavioral therapy (CBT) approach has been found to be helpful for female victims of rape but this was administered at least several weeks after the trauma. It has been suggested that CBT may be helpful if treating PTSD symptoms after a disaster event and may reduce the risk of long-term PTSD. There is also some evidence that this technique may be useful in minimizing PTSD in individuals who suffered mild brain injury. Special training in the use of these techniques should be obtained and there still needs to be further research before this approach is utilized on a regular basis.

MEDICATIONS

The most conservative psychopharmacologic treatment, as described, would be to try to assure continued treatment of chronic psychiatric conditions with previously prescribed medication. Short-term use of standard medications for insomnia and medications for persistent severe anxiety or psychotic manifestations could be used according to clinical judgment. The precipitation of major depression or mania particularly in vulnerable individuals will require psychopharmacotherapy along with close observation and hospitalization as needed.

There is research in progress, which may establish the use of anticonvulsant/antikindling agents that exert their effects through inhibition of glutaminergic agents. There is also the possibility of reduction of hypothalamic-pituitary-adrenal (HPA) activation with cortisol, which might prevent PTSD. Increasing serotonergic activities with selective serotonin reuptake inhibitors (SSRIs) and other drugs is also under consideration. Propanolol as a beta-adrenergic antagonist may prove to be useful in blocking the potentiation of the consolidation of the traumatic memory trace. However, until this is established or there is proper setting for study, these are not yet standard treatment approaches.

SPECIAL ISSUES WITH BIOLOGICAL, CHEMICAL, AND NUCLEAR TERRORISM

Biological, chemical, or nuclear (or radiation) terrorism or the immediate threat of these types of attacks raises certain psychological and psychiatric issues that may need to be addressed by a psychiatric consultant. Because the effects of these agents is quite different than the usual effects of explosion, fire, earthquakes, and other weather events, there is understandably great fear and potential panic when they are looming threats. Although large numbers of people could be affected by such agents, it is also possible that only a relatively small number of people will be directly injured but there could be mass hysteria and panic. Also these agents can spread slowly and silently leading to such panic.

Chemical and some biological agents work directly on the central nervous system. On one hand, they may present as delirium or other symptoms resembling neurotoxic symptoms well known to psychiatrists, which could include extreme anxiety, agitation, depression, and psychosis. These might have to be distinguished from individuals who have not been affected by such agents but are having marked anxiety and panic because of contagious fears. Similarly, radiation effects can lead to immediate nausea and long-term effects of harm to pregnant mothers and children as well as increasing cancer risks. The possibility of these effects can also lead to mass hysteria and psychosomatic symptoms in unexposed individuals. Similarly, a biological event such as a pandemic flu could create such problems as well as raising the difficult decisions involved in isolating people. A psychiatric consultant can be extremely helpful in triage in all these situations because he or she would be knowledgeable and experienced in diagnosing and understanding anxiety and panic disorders as well as delirium and other organic conditions.

RISK COMMUNICATIONS

In a world of mass communications, impending threats, real or imaginary, are readily transmitted around the world. National media and local media as well as people who provide content for the Internet need advice by psychological consultants. Similarly, local politicians and hospital administrators who speak to the media should appreciate the delicate balance required to transmit truthful information to the public in order to protect them without precipitating mass hysteria and undue anxiety and panic in both adults and children. An informed C-L psychiatrist who knows the psychological implications as well as the medical threats may turn out to be the best person to assist in this educational process.

Death, Dying, and Bereavement

Many years ago, when one of us was a junior attending, Elizabeth Kubler-Ross came to give grand rounds on death and dying. She described her then groundbreaking work, defining the five steps involved in accepting death that was due to a terminal illness. They were denial and isolation, anger, bargaining, depression, and finally acceptance. She reported that 90% of her patients came to the acceptance stage before death. Dr. Kubler-Ross took questions after the first part of her talk, and she was asked why so many of her patients were able to reach acceptance, whereas many of us averaged only a 10% to 30% rate of success. She shrugged her shoulders and said she did not know the reason for this disparity. She then went on with her talk, which involved discussing several case vignettes. After I heard the following vignette, I understood the reason for the high percentage of patients reaching the acceptance stage with Dr. Kubler-Ross.

CASE VIGNETTE: THE DYING PATIENT WHO WAS READY TO TALK

An 18-year-old girl was dying of Hodgkin's lymphoma. She had spent some time talking with Dr. Kubler-Ross about her feelings, but was not yet in the acceptance stage. It was New Year's Eve and Dr. Kubler-Ross was with her husband preparing for a large social gathering that evening at their home. Just as she was putting things in the oven, a phone call was received from the hospital indicating the 18-year-old patient was "ready to talk." Dr. Kubler-Ross reported that she looked at her husband and he looked her and said, "of course you should go." She went to the hospital and missed most of her social gathering, but the young girl was able to relate personal meaningful things to her, which reflected a new acceptance of her terminal illness. She died shortly thereafter.

We now know that patients do not simply go through the five stages in a sequential manner. Rather, there is often a fluidity of variable defenses as one goes back and forth, sometimes being angry and sometimes beginning to bargain with God or oneself. The defense of denial can be a very powerful defense mechanism that is not used only by those who are vulnerable and fragile. Like other mechanisms, its purpose is to protect the psyche from overwhelming anxiety.

Patients will usually not "give up" a defense mechanism unless they get some psychological gratification that allows them to be less anxious than before. In psychotherapy, this gratification comes with entering into a meaningful dialogue with another person who cares. This allows the patient to ultimately give up a protective defense. Hence, it became clear that Dr. Kubler-Ross' patient knew that her therapist would be there for her and finally felt comfortable talking about her anticipated death.

TO TELL OR NOT TO TELL

Often C-L psychiatrists are called when treating doctors are struggling with the question of whether they should tell their patient that they have a terminal illness or because of some emotional reaction around the patient who learns of a fatal prognosis. This is usually a "red herring," meaning that it is another one of those situations that is not what it seems to be. Certainly, before the 1970s, doctors almost never told patients about their terminal prognosis. Then there was a revolution in medical training as students, for the first time, were taught about death and dying. The problem is that while many doctors knew what they wanted to tell their patients, they did not really know how to talk and listen to them about this important life stage. This is where the C-L psychiatrist often comes in. When you are called in for a consultation about a death and dying issue, do not assume anything.

While the patient is usually the primary object of the consultation, you must be thinking of the doctors, nurses, and family, as any or all of them may be influencing the issue at hand. If the question is really, "Should the patient be told?", then the next question should be "Told what?" Does it mean "told that they have cancer?" Does it mean "told about a terminal prognosis?" What does a terminal prognosis mean? Does it mean that the patient is expected to die within a short period of time without treatment or that treatment will or will not prolong his or her life? What will the quality of his or her life be? Most important, if there is an opinion as to whether the patient should be told, who has this opinion? Is it that of the doctor, the family, the nurses, or the patient?

Sometimes the family will not want the doctor to tell the patient about the extent or prognosis of the illness and sometimes the patient will not want the family to be told the truth. On occasion, we have seen both parties telling the doctor not to tell the other about the fact of a terminal illness.

In the 21st century, our ethical code and the inclination of most doctors is that the patient has a right to all information about his or her medical condition. Some might still argue that there should be exceptions if that information will do harm to the patient. It would then be incumbent on the person making that argument to have convincing proof to this point. If there were serious debate about such an issue, there is usually a hospital ethics committee to mediate such a situation. (The C-L psychiatrist should stick to the psychiatric issues and not try to be a fountain of medical ethics when functioning as the clinician.)

Listen to the Patient

In reality, the psychiatrist should not be the person to tell the patient about the nature of the illness or the prognosis. This should be done by the treating physician (sometimes with your help, as indicated in subsequent text). You should not be drawn into the situation of conveying this information and you should always be on guard not to do so inadvertently during a consultation. However, it is perfectly acceptable and a good technique to ask the patient what he or she knows about the nature of the illness and also what he or she has been told about the outlook or prognosis of the illness. Frequently, you will find that patients know that they have a terminal illness long before the medical team has decided to tell them. The patient may have more optimistic views about the possibility of beating the illness or surviving long term than what may be the expected outcome. This may or may not be "denial" of the reality. Denial becomes important when it interferes with the possibility of a meaningful treatment. It also may be important if a person is denying the reality of an illness and then making life decisions, which could hurt him or her or the family (e.g., a patient who is denying the fact of a life-threatening illness and is buying a new house that will create a hardship for his family). Keep in mind that a patient can be helped to understand that he or she has a serious incapacitating illness, even if he or she is not ready to accept that the illness has a very poor prognosis.

Perhaps the most important issue that you can ask the patient in these situations would be "what questions about your illness do you have for your doctor." It also can be very useful as a consultant to teach our medical and surgical colleagues to ask this question of their patients. When we are asked what they should tell the patient, we can show them how to ask this question on a periodic basis. We can teach them how to listen to their patients (preferably while sitting down at the bedside) and convey that they are prepared to understand their questions and provide answers as best they can.

Often a patient expresses a desire to know all the details about his or her illness and then later changes his or her mind. The physician has to be alert for a shift in the patient's equilibrium about this important subject. The first vignette in this chapter shows a shift in the direction of the patient who wants to talk more about the fatal nature of her illness. The following vignette shows quite the opposite shift.

CASE VIGNETTE: THE DOCTOR WHO CHANGED HIS MIND

The patient was a young physician who needed exploratory laparotomy. The possibility of a malignancy was very real. The evening before the surgery, the patient asked his surgeon to make him a promise. It was that no matter what was found during surgery, the surgeon would come to him after the surgery and tell him the full extent of the findings and the prognosis. In fact, he said that he would not sign the consent form unless this promise was given. The surgeon agreed. During surgery it was found that the patient had widespread metastasis that was inoperable, with a grave prognosis. The incision was closed after a brief exploration and, after the patient recovered from the anesthesia, the surgeon visited the patient. He sat down at the bedside and was prepared to discuss the grim findings. The patient, however, showed no interest in hearing the full story. He assumed that the lesion was taken care of and had no questions to ask the surgeon.

Being with the Patient

Every C-L psychiatrist should have the experience of following patients during the dying process. You will find that this can be a very gratifying, as well as a helpful and meaningful process, for the patient. Under ideal circumstances, it should be the loved ones—family and/or friends—who should share this time with the patient, but sometimes this situation is so emotional for them that they cannot tolerate the closeness at this stage. You may be able to help them be with their loved ones during this time or be there together. Of course, you, as a C-L psychiatrist, have other responsibilities and usually cannot spend the extended time that a family member might spend with a dying relative. However, regular visits, even if brief, can allow a connection to be made that will be extremely helpful and meaningful to the dying patient. Keep in mind also that there is an expanding body of evidence which demonstrates that a physician's attitude and communication skills play a crucial role in how well patients cope with bad news.

Another reason why the C-L psychiatrist must have first-hand clinical experience with this phase of life is because it is also your role to teach your medical and surgical colleagues how to be with a dying patient. Often our colleagues are very receptive to learning how to deal with the emotional aspects of this stage of life.

ROLE OF CULTURE AND RELIGION

Understanding cultural, religious, and ethnic customs will be helpful in the treatment and interaction with a patient who is dying as well as with the subsequent grieving of family and friends.

PSYCHOLOGICAL AND PHYSICAL ASPECTS OF WORKING WITH THE DYING PATIENT

Psychological Aspects of Dying

Be careful not to be caught up in your own identifications and feeling about dying. Although it is always good to monitor your own countertransference, those things that make you anxious or depressed about dying might not be impacting your patient. (They may not even have an impact on you when you are in that stage of life.) Some of the common psychological issues that may come up are listed and discussed in subsequent text. It is better to hear patients articulate their own concerns and then perhaps clarify, validate, or interpret these concerns, rather than tell the patient what he or she is probably feeling or question them about the things that others often feel in this situation.

Separation Anxiety and Loss

Because no one has ever experienced death and discussed it, the closest experience that most people connect with the anticipation of death is "separation." Patients may acutely feel that they are separating from loved ones. Those people who have never handled separation well as children can be expected to have more anxiety than those who have coped well with separations in the past. Some patients also may be feeling the loss of anticipated events (e.g., the weddings of children, grandchildren, etc.).

Being alone is particularly difficult for many people. When family, clergy, or you make a commitment to be with them at the end of life, this can be experienced as very supportive. "Staying in contact" can be important and, as such, even a minimal physical touch by the psychiatrist can be very meaningful to the patient. Certainly, regular visits, even if quite brief in time (but hopefully sitting at the bedside rather than standing), will convey that the patient is not being abandoned.

The idea of living on through other people surfaces here and, when appropriate, the patient may want to talk about such feelings. In this connection, patients often will discuss their offspring, not only in terms of passing on their genes, but also the influence that they have had upon them. We often talk to patients about how they may have influenced other people at work or in their personal lives, which makes them feel as if they will live on. On occasion, the patient will want to give a personal gift to the psychiatrist (e.g., an item of clothing, a valued book, etc.) with the idea that a part of them will live on in this manner.

Control, Self-determination, and Self-esteem

Usually when someone is ill, he or she tends to lose control of his or her life. The patient is at the whim of the staff and, under some circumstances, cannot even go to the bathroom when he or she wishes to do so. In an attempt to regain some control, the patient may make what appear to be inappropriate requests or refuse various aspects of his or her treatment and care. For example, some patients in pain may request high doses of pain medication, even if it might endanger their already foreshortened lives. Others may refuse pain medication because they want to maintain the clarity of their thinking as close to the end as possible. By listening to the patient's wishes and making every effort to grant reasonable requests, we can help the patient feel worthwhile and respected. Patients' wishes may seem strange, but, yet, they may be very important. For example, some patients want certain music to be played during their dying. Often patients will have very specific requests regarding how their body should be covered or handled after death, as well as preferences for burial and so forth.

There are other ways in which the dying patient's self-esteem may be maintained. Pictures may be placed at the bed-side that portray the patient in an earlier healthier period, sur-rounded by things that indicated something about the patient (e.g., surrounded by children, riding a motorcycle, playing sports, in their work outfit, at school, etc.). This evokes inter-est and respect from the staff, which can enhance self-esteem.

Strengthening Relationships with Loved Ones

Studies have shown that dying patients often feel very strongly about strengthening their relationships with loved ones. You may have the opportunity to encourage such contact. At times, families will take the lead and may require the help of the psychiatrist in bending the rules to allow them to visit off hours or bring in children or do something meaningful with the patient, such as play music and so forth. The patient may want to discuss end-of-life treatments with family members, and such discussions can bring them closer together.

You may find that the patient is struggling with the desire to "take care of unfinished business." Sometimes this means talk-ing about thoughts, feeling, and memories, not only with the psychiatrist but also with the family. This may include asking for or offering forgiveness for things that have happened in the past. In some cases, encouraging the patient to write to family members (especially children) can be very therapeutic. When the patient is alert and there is a longer timeline, he or she may want to make a written or tape-recorded diary for family members who are not nearby. This can be helpful to the patient who wants to "live on" with loved ones and it also can be helpful to family members in the grieving period.

Physical Aspects of Dying
Palliative Care

Palliative care is therapy that focuses on decreasing pain and suffering by providing treatments for relief of symptoms along with comfort and support. Palliative care often involves a team approach that utilizes the treating doctor, the family, other health care professionals including mental health specialists, social services, and the clergy. The goal of palliative care is to allow the highest quality of life possible.

Doctors and nurses should be well trained in the principles of palliative care. Some hospitals have specialists or teams dedicated to this aspect of medical care. As a C-L psychiatrist, you should be an advocate for the patient, if necessary, and be sure that appropriate steps are taken to relieve as much of the discomfort of the patient as is possible.

The overwhelming majority of patients should not have to die in pain. There should be adequate communication between the patient and the staff so that adequate pain control is ensured. When there are painful conditions, regular dosing of pain medication is preferred to pain medication "as needed." Patients and doctors need to understand that physical dependency on narcotics is not a concern with the dying patient. There may be times when the patient prefers not to have full pain control in order to have a clear sensorium to communicate with family and friends (or with the psychiatrist). You should be well versed in pain medications and adjunctive techniques to assist in pain control, such as deep breathing, self-hypnosis, guided imagery, meditation, and so forth (Chapter 14).

In the course of talking with the patient, you may become aware of other palliative care issues that need to be addressed. It is quite appropriate for you to act as a liaison to be sure that adequate medical orders are written and appropriate medical care is carried out to relieve the patient's suffering. Proper bowel care is a good illustration of one of these issues. Constipation is often a side effect of medication for pain and should not be considered a minor medical issue, because it may cause a great deal of distress. Seemingly minor things, such as skin care, toileting, and positioning of the patient, are not really minor at all. They are the essence of patient comfort and you should pay attention to the patient's concerns about them. Respiratory issues are essential and, at times, very difficult to deal with. Dyspnea is one of the most frightening experiences a person can have. The patient can be encouraged to use bedside oxygen, which should be available. The decision to intubate and to use artificial respiration is a subject that ideally has been addressed with the patient at an earlier stage, as part of a "do not resuscitate" (DNR) discussion.

This is a good place to remind the reader that a request to do a "capacity evaluation" on a very sick or dying patient should not be limited to the perceived problem (just as we would hope that the cardiologist called to evaluate a heart murmur also would deal with related cardiac problems). A simple capacity evaluation often leads to a decision to work on a range of end-of-life issues.

Identification and Other "Countertransference"

Often it takes a certain amount of clinical experience and/or life experience to be comfortable working with dying patients. It is such an essential part of being a C-L psychiatrist that it behooves you to go out of your way to work closely with several such patients who would benefit by such contact. This will make you much more effective in day-to-day consultation work when interacting with other physicians and nurses who may be struggling around issues that are related to a dying patient on their service. Medical staff will sometimes, without even realizing it, begin to marginalize a patient who is dying. On rounds, they may only discuss the patient in the hallway and may not even enter the room. This behavior may be rationalized because "the patient is dying and there is not much we can do." The real reason for this avoidance is more likely the difficulty that the health care providers may have in facing death. This reminds us of our own inadequacies and limitations as healers. It also brings us face to face with our own mortality and the recognition that eventually we must face the loss of loved ones. Seeing a dying patient may bring back the painful experience of the grief that you experienced when someone close to you died. One of us found it very difficult to work with older men dying of cancer for approximately 6 months after losing a father.

Most doctors are not experienced in how to be with a dying patient. For this reason, we strongly recommend that you reach out to colleagues with whom you may be sharing a dying patient. Offer to periodically meet with them, perhaps over a cup of coffee, for discussion and supervision. Tell them that this is an important skill that comes with practice and guidance. Ask them to present a few minutes of process (the exact words of "she said, I said, etc.") of some interactions during their day-to-day work with the patient. Encourage them to spend a few minutes sitting down with the patient most days and to present that interaction to you for discussion. You, of course, will draw upon your experience as C-L psychiatrist who has closely worked with dying patients. Usually, it will be quite easy to make supportive recommendations that will help your colleagues understand their patients and be more effective in being with the dying patient. Do not underestimate the receptivity of even busy colleagues to your willingness to work with them in this area.

This offer of "supervision" or "discussion" around a case should not be limited to helping physicians. Nurses are usually the persons who best get to know the patients on a day-to-day basis. Many are very skilled and empathic in working with dying patients and their families, but, nevertheless, a similar offer of being a supervisor or a "sounding board" often will be very appreciated. The same holds true for social workers. Such investment of your time often will pay big dividends in having a good relationship with these colleagues around other patients. Sometimes we will learn a great deal ourselves from the interactions of our colleagues in these difficult situations. The following case shows how a junior colleague was able to use his life experience and insight to handle a very difficult situation.

CASE VIGNETTE: THE EMPATHIC RESIDENT

A male patient in his 30s with multiple traumas did not survive a motor vehicle accident and died in the emergency room (ER). The mother of the patient become hysterical and out of control. Nobody could calm her down. The first year (PGY-1) medical ER resident was the only one to stay in the room with her while she screamed and berated the hospital, the doctors, and the medical system. After he patiently stayed with her during the tirade, he gently asked her if there was anything he could do for her. She said, "Yes, remove the damn tube from his mouth" (endotracheal tube from her son). While he knew this was not usually the procedure because of the preference of the medical examiner, he did so in her presence and then turned to her and asked her if she would like to help him clean up the body. She agreed to do so and he asked the nurse for a basin of water and allowed her to clean her son's face. He stayed with her until she was ready to leave. When asked later by the C-L staff how he felt and how he was able to do this, he told the following story. Recently, his best friend had died. In his own subsequent grieving, he repeatedly thought of how painful it was for his friend's mother and how he had imagined such a loss would affect his own mother. He also recalled how his friend's mother said many times that she was bothered by seeing the tube in her son's mouth after he died. After the current ER incident, the resident was concerned that he did the wrong thing, especially in removing the tube. He was relieved when told by the C-L staff that he had handled the situation very well and seemed even more comfortable when we praised him to the director of training of the medical residency who then reaffirmed that he had done a good job.

BEREAVEMENT

Bereavement is the period of grief and mourning after a death. It is part of the normal process of reacting to a loss. The C-L psychiatrist has often had interaction with family and friends of the dying patient and may have been involved in the death notification process. In most cases, however, it is the responsibility of the treating physician to inform the family of the death of the patient. You should be aware that different religions and cultures have rituals and customs that are very important to the people involved. The grieving person may experience anger, guilt, anxiety, sadness, and despair. It is not unusual shortly after the death of a loved one for a person to hear their voice, which may actually be a hallucination, or to even have fleeting visual hallucinations of the deceased person. Symptoms can include sleeping problems, changes in appetite, or physical symptoms which may be an identification with the lost person or actual exacerbation of their own illness. It is common for even the well-adjusted grieving person to have episodes of tearfulness or crying whenever they are reminded of the loss. This may be accompanied by a deep abdominal sensation and some mild dyspnea, which have been described "as coming in waves." This response can be fairly powerful especially in the weeks and months after the loss. The duration of bereavement and intense grieving is variable and cannot be easily predicted. It can exist for at least 1 year.

LIAISON POTENTIAL

1. Of the inpatient services, the best place to connect in the role of a C-L psychiatrist and work regularly with staff

around patients who are dying would be on an oncology service.

2. Other units where there are ample clinical opportunities to work with dying patients and their families include intensive care units, burn units, and human immunodeficiency virus (HIV) units.

3. An on-call arrangement with the ER of the hospital also could provide an opportunity to see such patients and their families at the time of sudden death, as well as interact with staff who would benefit by being trained in this area.

4. A palliative care service or team would be another ideal place for a C-L psychiatrist to work with terminally ill patients.

5. Hospice programs provide an excellent setting for a psychiatrist who is interested in working with dying patients.

Appendix

Internet Websites Related to Each Chapter of this Book

The authors would like to thank Dr. George Alarado who was a medical student at New York Medical College for his assistance in compiling this list for the first edtion and Mr. Khan Fakhar a New York Medical College medical student for his assistance in revising the Web site list for this second edition.

THESE WEBSITES ARE A GOOD REFERENCE FOR TOPICS PRESENTED IN ALL CHAPTERS

American Psychiatric Association
http://www.psych.org/
American Psychological Association
http://www.apa.org
National Institute of Mental Health
http://www.nimh.nih.gov

CHAPTER 1—PRINCIPLES OF CONSULTATION-LIAISON PSYCHIATRY

Introduction

Academy of Psychosomatic Medicine

Onsite information about C-L Practice and residency guidelines. Linked to *Psychosomatics*, online journal of C-L psychiatry.
http://www.apm.org/

Psychiatric Disorders

Internet Mental Health

Information about different psychiatric disorders with links related to Internet sites.
http://www.mentalhealth.com/fr20.html

Psychology Self-Help Resources on the Internet

Listing of links pertaining to various mental disorders.
http://www.psywww.com/resource/selfhelp.htm

Karolinska Institute

Another collection of links pertaining to mental disorders.
http://www.mic.ki.se/Diseases/f3.html

CHAPTER 2—PSYCHOCARDIOLOGY
American Heart Association

Lay site with section for professionals. Searchable for anxiety, depression, and related to heart disease.
http://www.americanheart.org

Psychosomatics

Article discussing psychological factors and heart disease.
http://psy.psychiatryonline.org/cgi/content/full/41/4/372

Archives of Internal Medicine

Article on psychological factors and heart failure; plus links to related articles.
http://archinte.ama-assn.org/cgi/content/abstract/162/5/509

CHAPTER 3—PSYCHOONCOLOGY
Anxiety and Depression
National Cancer Institute

Description of the causes and treatment of anxiety experienced by cancer patients.
http://www.cancer.gov/cancertopics/pdq/supportivecare/anxiety/patient

International Union Against Cancer (UICC) World Cancer Congress

Psychiatric treatments: overview and effectiveness.
http://2006.confex.com/uicc/uicc/techprogram/P842.HTM

American Cancer Society

Link to "Coping with Cancer" section. Searchable, with sections for patients and professionals.
http://www.cancer.org/docroot/mbc/mbc_4x_anxiety
.asp?sitearea=mbc&level=1

Pain Management
International Psycho-Oncology Society

Provides many links to information on support groups and pain management for cancer patients.
http://www.ipos-society.org/survivors/links/pain.htm

Smoking
Medline Plus

Information on smoking cessation.
http://www.nlm.nih.gov/medlineplus/smokingcessation.html

CHAPTER 4—PSYCHONEPHROLOGY
Kidney Disorders
Kidney Patient News

Links to many kidney disease groups' websites.
http://www.kidneypatientnews.org/links.html

Medline Plus

End stage renal disease information.
http://www.nlm.nih.gov/medlineplus/ency/article/000500
.htm

National Kidney Foundation

General information about kidney disorders.
http://www.kidney.org/kidneyDisease/

Promoting Excellence in End-of-Life Care

A website with links to information about end stage kidney disease and dialysis.

http://www.promotingexcellence.org/i4a/pages/Index
.cfm?pageID=3863

Dialysis
E-Medicine

Encephalopathy, dialysis.
http://www.emedicine.com/med/topic665.htm

CHAPTER 5—PSYCHOLOGICAL CARE OF THE BURN AND TRAUMA PATIENT
Burns
Medline Plus

Information on burns.
http://www.nlm.nih.gov/medlineplus/burns.html

Phoenix Society for Burn Victims

Website connecting burn survivors, their loved ones, and
burn care professionals with valuable resources.
http://www.phoenix-society.org/

Post-traumatic Stress Disorder
SAMHSAs National Mental Health Information Center

Website provides physicians with information to explore a
variety of roles in disaster response and recovery as well as
tools to better assess and treat the needs of their patients.
http://www.mentalhealth.samhsa.gov/publications/allpubs/
sma95-3022/default.asp

National Center for Post-traumatic Stress Disorder

Disaster Mental Health Services: A Guidebook for Clinicians
and Administrators: includes sections dealing with adults,
children, and psychopharmacology.
http://www.ncptsd.org/treatment/disaster/index.html

Fenichel's Current Topics in Psychology

Trauma resources; numerous links on various aspects of
trauma, with emphasis on 9/11.
http://www.fenichel.com/trauma.shtml

CHAPTER 6—PSYCHOLOGICAL CARE OF THE OBSTETRICS/GYNECOLOGY PATIENT
Women's Mental Health

A good reference website for all of the topics discussed in this chapter.
www.womensmentalhealth.org

Pregnancy and Postpartum Depression
Postpartum Depression

Many links for information on postpartum depression.
http://www.psycom.net/depression.central.post-partum.html

e-Medicine

Information on hyperemesis gravidarum.
http://www.emedicine.com/emerg/topic479.htm

Psychiatric Times

Article on psychiatric disorders during pregnancy.
http://www.psychiatrictimes.com/p030117.html

CHAPTER 7—PSYCHIATRIC ASPECTS OF WOMEN'S HEALTH
Women's Mental Health

A good reference website for all of the topics discussed in this chapter.
www.womensmentalhealth.org

CHAPTER 8—PSYCHIATRIC ASPECTS OF GASTROENTEROLOGY
Peptic Ulcers
Intellihealth

Search for stress and peptic ulcers.
http://www.intellihealth.com/IH/ihtIH/EMIHC000/24479/21923/253296.html?d=dmtSimple

Irritable Bowel Syndrome
About Irritable Bowel Syndrome

Neurobiology of stress and emotions related to irritable bowel
   syndrome.
http://www.aboutibs.org/publications/stress.html

Liver Disease
Merck Manual

Alcoholic liver disease.
http://www.merck.com/pubs/mmanual/section4/chapter40/
   40a.htm

Eating Disorders
National Eating Disorders Association

Eating Disorders Information Index
http://www.nationaleatingdisorders.org/
   p.asp?webpage_ID=294

CHAPTER 9—PSYCHIATRIC ASPECTS OF ENDOCRINOLOGY AND AUTOIMMUNE DISORDERS
Thyroid Disease
Medline Plus

Thyroid disorders.
http://www.nlm.nih.gov/medlineplus/thyroiddiseases.html

Thyroid Information

Search for depression, related topics.
http://www.thyroid-info.com/articles/cohendepression.htm

Diabetes
American Diabetes Association

"For Professionals" section with access to relevant journals.
   Searchable.
http://www.diabetes.org/home.jsp

National Institute of Diabetes, Digestive, and Kidney Disorders

Search for psychology, depression, and so on.
http://www.niddk.nih.gov

Chronic Fatigue Syndrome and Fibromyalgia
Medline Plus

Chronic fatigue syndrome.
http://www.nlm.nih.gov/medlineplus/
   chronicfatiguesyndrome.html

Chronic Fatigue Syndrome and Fibromyalgia Forum

http://www.co-cure.org/

Systemic Lupus Erythematosus
Lupus Foundation of America

Depression in lupus information.
http://www.lupus.org/education/brochures/depress07.html

CHAPTER 10—PSYCHIATRIC ASPECTS OF NEUROLOGIC DISORDERS
Stroke
National Stroke Association

Lay site with section for professionals.
http://www.stroke.org/

TSAO Foundation

For caregivers; coping with psychology of stroke patients.
http://www.tsaofoundation.org/caregivers/stroke06.html

Dementia
Medline Plus

Dementia
http://www.nlm.nih.gov/medlineplus/dementia.html

Neurology Channel

Dementia
http://www.neurologychannel.com/dementia/index.shtml

Multiple Sclerosis
UCSF Multiple Sclerosis Center

Health psychology of multiple sclerosis.
http://mscenter.ucsf.edu/psychology.htm#health_psychology

CHAPTER 11—PSYCHIATRIC ASPECTS OF SURGERY AND TRANSPLANTATION
American Society of Plastic Surgeons

Psychological aspects of plastic surgery.
http://www.plasticsurgery.org/public_education/procedures/
  psychological_aspects.cfm

e Medicine

Psychological aspects of plastic surgery.
http://www.emedicine.com/ent/topic36.htm

Critical Care Nurse

Psychiatric aspects of transplantation.
http://www.aacn.org/aacn/jrnlccn.nsf/
  c54ad59fdf5d6228882565a0006a1369/
  895f91ba7ae85fe3882567830071110f?OpenDocument

Psychosomatic Medicine

Hemodynamic and emotional responses to a psychological
  stressor after cardiac transplantation.
http://www.psychosomaticmedicine.org/cgi/content/full/63/
  2/289

Medscape

Psychological aspects of transplantation.
http://www.medscape.com/viewarticle/436541_print

Virginia Commonwealth University

Psychological assessment and care of organ transplant
  patients.
http://www.vcu.edu/psych/files/JCCP%202002.pdf

CHAPTER 12—HUMAN IMMUNODEFICIENCY VIRUS/ACQUIRED IMMUNODEFICIENCY SYNDROME PSYCHIATRY

Human Immunodeficiency Virus and Acquired Immunodeficiency Syndrome

Human Immunodeficiency Virus Clinical Resource—New York State Acquired Immunodeficiency Syndrome Institute

www.hivguidelines.org

Johns Hopkins Acquired Immunodeficieny Syndrome Service

Information on epidemiology, prevention, practice guidelines, as well as related links.
http://www.hopkins-aids.edu

Center for Disease Control

Topics covered include basic science, surveillance, vaccine resources, and prevention tools.
http://www.cdc.gov/hiv/dhap.htm

AIDSMEDS.COM

Depression and HIV.
http://www.aidsmeds.com/lessons/Depression1.htm

CHAPTER 13—SOMATOFORM DISORDERS, FACTITIOUS DISORDERS, AND MALINGERING

Somatization Disorder

American Academy of Family Physicians

Practical diagnosis of somatization.
http://www.aafp.org/afp/20000215/1073.html

Medline Plus

About somatization disorder.
http://www.nlm.nih.gov/medlineplus/ency/article/000955.htm

e Medicine

Somatization disorder.
http://www.emedicine.com/ped/topic3015.htm

Factitious Disorder
Merck Manual

Factitious disorder (Munchausen's).
http://www.merck.com/pubs/mmanual/section15/
  chapter185/185d.htm

e Medicine

About factitious disorder.
http://www.emedicine.com/MED/topic3125.htm

CHAPTER 14—PAIN MANAGEMENT
Pain Management
National Pain Education Council

Information about the clinical management of pain; free
  registration.
http://www.npecweb.org/

American College of Physicians-American Society of Internal Medicine

Ten questions to identify drug-seeking patients.
http://www.acponline.org/journals/news/apr02/drug_seeking
  .htm

American Academy of Pain Management

http://www.aapainmanage.org/

Pain.com

http://www.pain.com

American Pain Foundation

http://www.painfoundation.org/

Beth Israel Department of Pain Medicine and Palliative Care

http://www.stoppain.org/

American Academy of Pain Medicine

Good list of Internet resources.
http://www.painmed.org/

CHAPTER 15—CAPACITY DETERMINATION
Capacity and Informed Consent
American Academy of Family Physicians

Evaluating patient capacity in practice.
http://www.aafp.org/afp/20010715/299.html

Wikipedia

Informed consent.
http://en.wikipedia.org/wiki/Informed_consent

Northwestern—Legal Issues

Medical decision capacity.
http://endlink.lurie.northwestern.edu/legal_issues/capacity
.cfm

American Medical Association

Informed consent.
http://www.ama-assn.org/ama/pub/category/4608.html

CHAPTER 16—PSYCHODYNAMIC ISSUES AND PSYCHOTHERAPY IN THE CONSULTATION-LIASION SETTING
Psychotherapy
The Royal College of Psychiatrists

Types of psychotherapy.
http://www.rcpsych.ac.uk/mentalhealthinformation/
therapies/psychotherapy.aspx

PsychNet—United Kingdom

Directory of psychotherapy links (four pages total).
http://www.psychnet-uk.com/psychotherapy/psychotherapy_
general1.htm#psychotherapy

CHAPTER 17—SUBSTANCE ABUSE ISSUES IN THE MEDICAL SETTING

Substance Abuse

Prevline

SAMHSA's National Clearinghouse for information on alcohol and drugs.

http://www.health.org/

Medline Plus

Substance abuse.

http://www.nlm.nih.gov/medlineplus/substanceabuse.html

American Academy of Addiction Psychiatry

http://www.aaap.org/

Med Bio World

Listing of useful links regarding substance abuse.

http://www.sciencekomm.at/med/assoc/addiction.html

CHAPTER 18—DISASTER PSYCHIATRY

New Resources and Materials

Church Disaster Mental Health Project

This website provides active outreach and education to pastors and church leaders regarding disaster response and recovery.

http://www.churchdisasterhelp.org/index.html

Special Populations: Emergency and Disaster Preparedness

This National Library of Medicine web page provides links to selected websites featuring emergency preparedness for special populations, including people with disabilities, older adults, children, and women.

http://sis.nlm.nih.gov/outreach/
specialpopulationsanddisasters.html

Research Education Disaster Mental Health (REDMH)

The website provides research summaries, instructional materials, information on REDMH mentoring programs, and resources for disaster mental health researchers.

http://www.redmh.org/index.html

The National Survey on Drug Use and Health Report: Impact of Hurricanes Katrina and Rita on Substance Use and Mental Health

This special issue presents two analyses related to the prevalence of substance use and mental health issues before and after Hurricanes Katrina and Rita in the gulf State disaster area.

http://download.ncadi.samhsa.gov/prevline/pdfs/NSDUH08-0131.pdf

The British Journal of Psychiatry

Biochemical terrorism.
http://bjp.rcpsych.org/cgi/content/full/183/6/491

Yale University
Bioterrorism resources.
http://info.med.yale.edu/library/subjects/bioterrorism.html

Disaster Psychiatry Outreach

Links to several educational resources.
http://www.disasterpsych.org/Default.aspx?PageID=10

CHAPTER 19—DEATH, DYING, AND BEREAVEMENT
End-of-Life Care
Growth House

Information and resource on end-of-life care.
http://www.growthhouse.org/

Center to Advance Palliative Care

Last Acts is a campaign to improve end-of-life care by a coalition of professional and consumer organizations with excellent search capacity in palliative care and other related topics.
http://www.lastacts.com

Medline Plus

Search for "death and dying."
http://www.nlm.nih.gov/medlineplus/

Index